HOW TO MAKE
GREAT LOVE
TO A WOMAN

Also by Anne Hooper and Phillip Hodson

How to Make Great Love to a Man

HOW TO MAKE
GREAT LOVE
TO A WOMAN

ANNE HOOPER AND PHILLIP HODSON

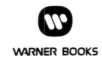

WARNER BOOKS

An AOL Time Warner Company

Warner Books Edition

This Warner Books edition is published by arrangement with
Robson Books, 10 Blenheim Court, Brewery Road, London N7 9NT

Visit our Web site at www.twbookmark.com.

 An AOL Time Warner Company

Printed in Canada
Originally published in hardcover by Robson Books
First Warner Books Printing: June 2002
10 9 8 7 6 5 4 3 2 1

Library of Congress Cataloging-in-Publication Data

Hooper, Anne
    How to make great love to a woman / Anne Hooper and Phillip Hodson.—Warner Books ed.
        p. cm.
    Originally published: London : Robson Books, 2000.
    Includes bibliographical references.
    ISBN 0-446-67834-1
    1. Sex instruction for men. 2. Men—Sexual behavior. 3. Women-Physiology. 4.
Communication in sex. I. Hodson, Phillip, II. Title.

HQ36 .H66 2002
613.9'6—dc21

                                                                    2001046554

Photography by John Freeman
Art Direction and Styling by Jack Buchan
Illustrations by Stuart Miller

contents

Preface

Most people might think that, when you are asked to write two books on sex, one for men and another for women, all you have to do is change every 'him' for 'her' then one book becomes two. An economy of words and good husbandry of text, a quick trip round the writing factory to conserve vocabulary and we have covered the territory and managed to be equitable in the process.

Except that sex, and men and women, aren't like that. As joint authors we feel strongly that each gender has very different sexual needs and desires. If this book and its companion *How to Make Great Love to a Man* are going to possess any real meaning, this must be reflected in how they are written. Not a lot of point in banging on about love, romance and tenderness if all the male readers really want is the 'hard stuff'. Not a lot of point in describing 101 ways in which to do sex standing up if the female readers wouldn't dream of having sex without a few preliminaries – such as getting to know each other, trusting, falling in love and so on.

It's not that women can't be just as rough and tough in bed as men – they frequently *are*. Lots of women love quickies. Lots of women adore the frenzy when you can't wait to get your clothes off and you're in so much of a hurry that you do it against the living room wall or inside the office with the door locked or in the kitchen two minutes before the guests arrive. But they adore it because, in most cases, there is more to the relationship than just a 'knee-trembler'. If the quick bang were the *only* expression of love and sex, they wouldn't be quite so enthusiastic.

So our two books are deliberately written to be very different in approach. This book focuses on the emotional approach to good sex because that is what most women appreciate. It looks at all the factors that feed into a woman's mind so that she not only feels sexy, she is able *totally to let go with all her passion.*

HER SEXUAL BACKGROUND

Freud once said: 'When two people make love there are at least four people present'. He was talking about the fantasy lover or lovers who might be lurking in your mind. The bit he missed out is that shades of parents will be present too. Some of a woman's response will have been dictated by the warmth and sensuality of her upbringing. If her parents were repressive and cold, she may find it very hard to let go of inhibition. If her parents were warm and sensual, there shouldn't be too much difficulty.

There's a simple test that you can do based on early recollections. Find out what is her earliest memory of being touched lovingly? We're not talking sex here, just affection.

The answers can be surprising and often dismaying. One woman we know said she couldn't remember being touched lovingly by her parents *at all.* A male friend was never touched lovingly by his mother but fortunately his father made up for this during early childhood, showing his affection with hugs and attention. The right answer could be cuddles with your mother as a little tot, walking hand in hand or arm in arm as a child, being soaped in the bath, all innocent activities that let you feel someone loves you. It's this that forms the basis for your free and uninhibited expression of sexuality as an adult. Looking into such remote corners of your own and your partner's life can be a fascinating exercise. It can also make relating sensually easier to do.

LOVE IS WONDERFUL

Love plays a big part in sex for most women. We believe that it does for men too. Men depend on being loved, men fall in love more easily and out of love with greater difficulty than women. But men don't depend quite so much on the trappings of love, the romance, the flowers, the power of passionate suggestion as do women, for their actual turn on. Any sex book for women must include a serious chapter on how to let her *feel* loved, as this one does.

SEXY STORIES FOR WOMEN

There is a whole dimension to the thinking/feeling side of women's sexuality, which is hardly rated by men at all because, to them, it seems so low key. We are talking romantic erotica here. Women adore reading historical romances, they love sexy novels, they devour escapist fiction. Why? Because it provides them with a romance they may never experience in real life. But, also, because such literature turns them on. It's what we call the Mr D'Arcy factor. The sheer power of Mr D'Arcy's thighs as he squeezes his lucky horse between them, the damp ruffled shirt clinging to his powerful chest, 'phwoarr!' as most sane women would say. Bearing in mind that erotic fiction is known to heighten women's arousal (it's actually used during some sex therapy) we include a chapter where we publish our own short selection. Reading aloud is a friendly activity. If you read these short stories together you will, with any luck, grow considerably more than friendly.

FEELING SEXUALLY FREE

Although most men would like to be known by their friends as fearless and devastatingly attractive, we are well aware that the most brazen chaps still possess a few uncertainties tucked away at the back of the brain. Bearing man's real vulnerability in mind we end this book by celebrating an all time first for a sex manual. We include a chapter on appreciating life in general, as well as life in the bedroom, on the grounds that, even if a relationship doesn't work out, there is still a lot of living to do. Despite gloom and doom, it's a good idea to try and tune into life. The idea of using a mantra has, up till now, been dismissed as New Age nonsense. But mantras, when they function properly, work in the same way as positive thinking. A simple written mantra is just a natural tool for reminding the brain to appreciate life.

We've enlarged the mantra system here to include some specifically sexual ones. Just carrying a note in your wallet containing the words 'I AM FREE TO FEEL SENSUAL' can make you take (safe) decisions that you previously would have left alone. Pick the sentence you think good for you and copy it out. With any luck, this book actually will change your life!

Anne Hooper

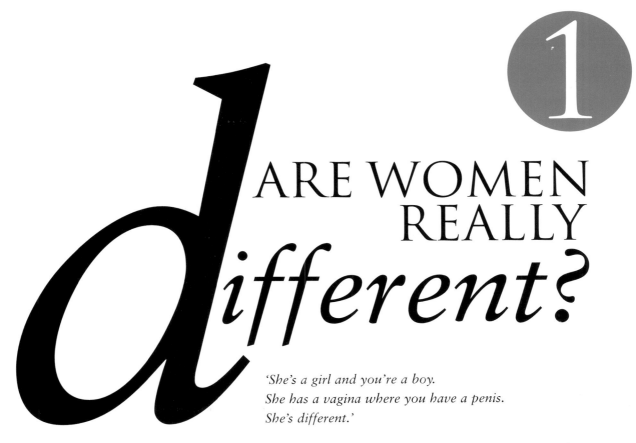

*d*ARE WOMEN REALLY *ifferent?*

'She's a girl and you're a boy.
She has a vagina where you have a penis.
She's different.'

This is the earliest explanation offered to small children in the first round of the Great Debate. You know the one – it's that 'Are women really aliens?' question. From the age of two, the Debate affects us all. History suggests that the controversy is continuous.

TWENTIETH CENTURY SEX WAR

❦ In the 1930s James Thurber published his cartoon narrative *The War Between the Sexes* where strange vitriolic women were pictured engulfing hapless, innocent men – *women were the enemy.*

❦ In the 1960s and 70s the pendulum was pushed so far in the opposite direction by the feminists as to force the question 'Are Men Really Necessary?' At the same time sex research charted, accurately for the first time, the journey of human sexual response. What astonished everyone who read the findings was that male and female sexual response turned out to be so *similar.*

❦ The convergence of sex research, feminism and the invention of the contraceptive pill added up in the mid-1970s to a new era in which the so-called Sexual Revolution took place. A characteristic of the Sexual Revolution was that, for the first time in history, women were allowed to be as sexually outgoing as men. *Men and women were equal.* This meant that, in theory, women were able to have as many sex partners as they liked, to invite sex, to enjoy casual sex, in short to behave sexually as men already had for years. Some of them did. A lot of them didn't. But the foundations for sexual equality were laid. Men benefited from this outgoing behaviour by, well, just getting more sex. For the time being, a truce was declared in the sex war.

- In the 1980s AIDS brought much sexual experimentation to a halt and *the sexes recouped*, falling back on more exclusive dating and mating patterns but still bringing the idea of equality into the bedroom and into relationships.

- The 1990s emerged from the blanket of monogamy to examine the fact that, whichever way you enjoy sex, *women's actual relationships with men didn't come up to scratch.* Women voted, with their feet, to maintain their own separate households, not always to live with their male and not only to have his children.

Clinical researcher John Gottman and writer John Gray are the latest contributors to the Debate:

- the former declares that men can't deal with emotional flooding, which probably means that women shouldn't confront them (heaven for the chaps but hell for the women);

- the latter teaches that the differences between men and women are so great that they are effectively from different planets (a recipe, we suggest, for giving up).

Serious research into sex difference has been taking place for decades but, in the past 20 years, has speeded up. We understand a lot more about sexual diversity than we used to but the Debate still hasn't resolved the Nature versus Nurture argument, ie. what causes such diversity? That's probably because the evidence shows that both biology *and* social learning are important to the shaping of our sexuality. Almost certainly, each interrelates with the other. This makes understanding complicated. Today, in the third millennium, genetic research takes us on to yet another round of scientific information.

HOW WE DIFFER – 1

The theory, therefore, goes that men with higher testosterone levels tend to carry the competitive behaviour associated with testosterone and dominance into relationships with the opposite sex. The logical deduction from this is that women, possessing a much lesser degree of testosterone in their make up, have less need to dominate and, as a result, are much easier to live with.

NATURE

The biological theory has highlighted the role of sex hormones and how these affect the development of physiological characteristics with the additional likelihood that they *also influence emotions*. John Money and colleagues of Johns Hopkins University, Baltimore have made a life study of patients, young and old, who have been subjected to unusual hormonal exposure and it is from these patients that Money developed his seminal theories.

There is his work, for example, with androgenised women. These are women who, by virtue of genetic error or drugs their mothers received during pregnancy, were exposed to an excess of androgen during their foetal development. In outward appearance these individuals appear male. Their genitals may look like anything between an enlarged clitoris to an undeveloped penis. *Yet, these are girl children.*

The medical treatment, developed by Money, is to feminize the genitals, shortly after birth and if necessary to dose with an androgen (testosterone) suppressant. The really interesting part is when adolescence and adulthood are reached. Money reports distinct differences in behaviour between these and ordinary women. The androgenised group were less interested in stereotypical female roles, less interested in caring for children and more likely to give priority to a career. They were also more outgoing, more outwardly active, with preferences for male interests and clothes.

Money's theory is that hormones programme the brain and that behaviour is duly affected. Research in the 1990s on 4,500 US army veterans by Alan Booth and James Dabbs of Penn and Georgia State Universities appears to back this up and shows that men producing more testosterone were less likely to marry and more likely to divorce. It was only those with a relatively low level of testosterone who were likely to report marital success.

THE GENES HAVE IT

In recent years research has discovered specific differences in the way male and female brains are organised. Psychologist Daniel Goleman reports a finding that the two halves of the brain appear to be arranged differently with more specialisation likely for men and better socialisation for women. Later work with Asperger's Syndrome (a form of autism) backs this up – the majority of sufferers are men.

SPECIFIC SEX DIFFERENCES

In an extensive survey of the work on this subject there appear to be four distinct differences that emerge.

1   There is strong evidence that males are more aggressive than females. This becomes apparent by the age of two and a half and is observed in all cultures.

2   Boys have more visual spatial ability than girls.

3   Boys appear to be better at mathematics.

4   Girls appear to be better at verbal tasks and possess more adept verbal skills. This last is controversial since there are several studies disproving this but most recently a large study seemed to show that little girls possessed many more hundreds of words in their vocabulary than boys of the equivalent age. Interestingly, work with brain-damaged individuals showed that the women were less severely impaired verbally than the men, regardless of where in the brain the damage actually occurred.

ALL THOUGHT – LITTLE EMOTION

Asperger's Syndrome is characterised by an inability to relate to emotions, and a preference for interpreting the world through thought. Asperger's men can become wonderful engineers and architects. But they can be extremely difficult to be married to since they possess no 'instinctive' understanding of what a wife is feeling. There is a growing belief that there may be many thousands of seemingly ordinary men who suffer from Asperger's syndrome to some degree, accounting for much of 'the war between the sexes'.

Syndromes such as Asperger's are the result of genetic inheritance. Science now recognises that many such syndromes are sex-linked, with the anomalous gene switched on in one sex but switched off in the other. Asperger's is 10 times more common in boys than it is in girls. In Turners syndrome (where one of the X chromosomes is missing from the normal XX female makeup), the sufferer is 400 times more likely to inherit the gene from their mother. Scientists now believe that the male brain typically processes spatial information and understanding of physical systems – the female brain possesses better ability to read human faces and has greater aptitude for social reasoning. Genetic science classifies Asperger's as being an extreme point of the male brain continuum.

NURTURE

If the entire way in which we relate is laid down in the genes, what is the point, you may ask, of doing anything but throwing your hands up in the air and screaming 'forget it'? The answer is that, even though the brain lays down a blue-print, our upbringing, the education we receive as children, formally or informally, also plays its part. This is Nurture.

There have been innumerable studies that demonstrate that adults react to children differently depending on whether they 'believe' they are male or female. And at around the age of 18 months, says Money, our *own* beliefs about gender take over. If we think we are male, we unconsciously adopt the appropriate role. The same is true for girls.

BRAIN RESEARCH

Daniel Goleman in his book *Emotional Intelligence* describes the research work of Richard Davidson, a University of Wisconsin psychologist. Davidson has discovered that people with a history of clinical depression have lower levels of brain activity in the left frontal lobe and more on the right than did people who had never been depressed. Using this knowledge, Davidson was also able to predict with children as young as 10 months old with 100 per cent precision, which ones would cry when their parents left them alone for a while in a strange room.

Why describe something which seems so unrelated to sex? Well, even though babies may be born with such brain differences, the good news from scientist Jerome Kagan of Harvard is that with the right firm training from our mothers we can learn to change such behaviour. And that although this gets harder with age, *the brain continues to shape itself and be shaped throughout life*. Nor do we suddenly stop at the age of 20, never developing any further.

Why does this matter to readers simply wanting to know more about giving their woman a wonderful time in bed? By understanding such differences we get a handle on them. We gain in optimism. This means that, if something goes wrong between two people, we can learn to alter behaviour so that things get the optimum chance of going right again. It means that if an emotional difficulty interferes with sexual expression, there are ways of learning to overcome it. It also means that even when things go amazingly well in our love lives, there is the wonderful thought they can continue to be enhanced.

What about the specific sex differences, though? How and where do these show up? Do they matter? Can they be modified so that our partners love us more or less? Will we be able to induce a partner to change, should we feel the necessity strongly?

WHAT ABOUT SEX?

Research into the nuts and bolts of sex shows that most physical aspects of sexual response in men and women are similar. We experience the same stages of sexual arousal, and when enjoying climaxes do so with exactly the same time interval of orgasmic contractions (0.8 per second!). However, where woman differ is that some of them are capable of experiencing routine multiple orgasm. According to therapists Hartman and Fithian, so too are men, but this appears to require youth, special training and a prior agreement on definitions.

For years, many dyed-in-the-wool medical men protested that women could not experience orgasm because they didn't experience ejaculation. However much you might try to explain that there are differences between orgasm and ejaculation, this was the line persistently taken. Imagine the dismay of such medical fogeys when the news about G-spot ejaculation was announced. (More in Chapter Six). Although only a minority of women experience it, ejaculation is triggered from a spot on the anterior wall of the vagina. The theory goes that this spot may be the vestige of what would have developed into a prostate gland, should the foetus have turned into a boy at around the sixth week of pregnancy, instead of a girl.

FETISHES

One specific sex difference however lies in the area of sexual fetish. Men are far more likely to be exhibitionists, fetishists and paedophiles. Men appear to be turned on by parts of women, such as their legs, their feet, even their high-heeled shoes. Men can become seriously attached to rubber aprons, wellington boots, shiny polythene, finding it increasingly difficult to climax without the assistance of these objects. Research also shows us a few men who are compulsively and destructively fetishistic and who are also violent, self-destructive and likely to possess a criminal record. Women of this type are rare.

PORNOGRAPHY AND MEN

One of the current and distressed complaints made by many women is that their men appear to spend more time being turned on by sex magazines than by their partners. Presumably some men *may* be making a specific choice to be unfaithful to a wife with a photographic model. It's our contention, however, that many of the men seduced by porn may not be making any such logical decision. We may be hearing that these guys, displaying a mildly fetishistic behaviour, as Gosselin and Wilson describe it, are also motivated by genuine brain differences.

SEXUAL DEVELOPMENT IN THE WOMB

For those not in the know, all foetuses start off female and it is only when the Y chromosome inherited from the father comes into active play that the male foetus is bathed in androgen around the sixth week which then causes it to develop male characteristics. The foetus XX, destined to be a girl, simply carries on developing with no change of direction. This may explain why boys are more fragile, more vulnerable than girls – they have had to endure major change when so immature.

PSYCHOLOGY OF FETISHISM

In their book *Sexual Variations* (1980) Drs Chris Gosselin and Glenn Wilson of the Institute of Psychiatry say:

❦ Fetishists tend to be more introverted than conventional people

❦ Introverts are more easily conditioned than extroverts; they're more sensitive to stimuli and acquire emotional associations more powerfully

❦ They are therefore more likely to turn on to *any* sexual association

If fetishistic behaviour is a matter of learning, why is it that *women* don't learn it as easily as men? The answer goes:

1 Psychological studies show that men are more sensitive to visual stimuli than women. They are more likely to pick up and focus on some eye-catching object.

2 Much initial learning seems to follow the model of classic conditioning. In this case, men see the object and are then given a pleasurable stimulus that they later associate with the object. The object and the eroticism are paired. Men's genitals, the penis in particular, play a more prominent part in early erotic life than do women's genitals. It is the association (the biofeedback) of the penis and object which make the first connections.

3 Arousal is a third key part to the process. Gosselin and Wilson say that arousal need not be directly sexual at all but just the general state of being awake or aware: 'To some extent the body, as opposed to the mind, has difficulty in distinguishing one form of arousal from another; as a result, any strong emotion can be translated in the mind, under appropriate conditions, into sexual arousal. Some famous experiments by Stanley Schacter of Stanford University have shown that the effects of adrenalin – a general stimulant – may be described by subjects as fear, anger, or even love … '

WHAT IS THE SOLUTION?

❦ First, for both partners to understand what is happening.

❦ Second, for the male to attempt to show extra love for his partner, increased sexual attention and much more discretion about his private activities.

❦ Third, for the female to get it clear in her head that everyone is entitled to a private life and that she does not own her husband's body. If a partnership is to remain equitable she certainly needs to feel she is getting her fair erotic share but provided this is the case, she equally needs to be tolerant.

If we return to Asperger's Syndrome, we remember that Asperger's type characteristics are the far end of a *normal* spectrum of male behaviour. Many men therefore may not see the emotional connection their wives are making between porn and jealousy because their own particular brain make-up is not constructed to make that same emotional connection. For them this would not be logical, as Mr Spock would say. Perhaps these same men instead dismiss their wives' distress as irrational.

This explanation is emphatically not to condone such male behaviour. If you truly want to make things work with your woman, if you sincerely

want her to have a fantastic sex life with you, we feel you must learn to appreciate such connections for your own sake, as well as for hers.

SEX BOREDOM

Dr Glenn Wilson stated in 1989 that there is 'one 'disorder of desire' that affects men more strikingly than women – the boredom that arises from repetitive sex with the same partner'. Wilson is a biological, anthropological psychologist who believes that the 'need for periodic recharging of libido (in men) by novel females that is seen in most mammals is a ... manifestation of the males' reproductively optimal 'promiscuity strategy'.'

He is dismissive of the problem this throws up since he states that the disorder is 'not a disease but a normal biological phenomenon based on natural sex differences'. That's as maybe but 1999 findings on testosterone levels seem to show that it's the fellas with *not* so much of the stuff coursing through their veins that make the best, most long-term husbands. Perhaps there is an answer but one that men won't like – which is to dampen down testosterone with a chemical antidote. Anyone for bromide?

FEMALE PASSIVITY

Another difference, induced by Nurture, is that women have been expected to be the more passive of the two sexes and, as a result, have shaped their behaviour accordingly. This means that they wait to be asked out on a date, wait for the man to make the first physical move, expect him to know what to do in bed. Or it used to mean this. Thanks to feminist teaching of the 70s and 80s, women (and men) in therapy groups have been slowly revising these expectations. Fewer women of the younger generations would expect to behave like this today. But attitudes take time to change.

One of these teaching methods is that of assertion technique. This proved vital to some women who were so accustomed to regarding a partner's choice as their own that they had to be taught how to make choices that concerned only them. You, as a man, might think it desirable that your woman should think only of you. But, interestingly enough, it can become irritating. Her total acquiescence sometimes gives the appearance of having no character, no mind of her own. But everyone has a character – lurking there, somewhere underneath. One participant in a group told the other women: 'I never climax but this doesn't

THE YES/NO EXERCISE

In one week:

❦ Say YES to three things you really want to do

❦ Say NO to three things you really don't want to do.

The object of the exercise is to practise being assertive instead of giving in passively and to determine what your priorities actually consist of. You can say YES to something as mundane as eating a rich chocolate bar or you can say YES to something that is so major it is life-changing. One pupil stunned her group by revealing she had packed in her boyfriend because she didn't really like him, packed in her job and set up a freelance business and changed her flat because she didn't like her flatmates. All this on the strength of deciding to say Yes or No!

TELEPHONE DATING

One telephone survey carried out at the beginning of the 1990s found that women believed that their man would think badly of them if they telephoned him to ask for a first date whereas the men said that they would love the women to do so and would think highly of them for calling. Such women callers needed to learn courage.

matter because I feel so happy for my husband when he has his.' She honestly thought her lack of sexual response didn't matter. But it did. And most of all, it mattered to her – even if she didn't acknowledge it.

What can you do to assist such a hard case? You can start off by teaching her a simple assertion exercise. We wish we had bought shares in this exercise some 25 years ago because we never seem to stop writing or teaching about it.

DIFFERENCES OF SEX DRIVE

The hormone testosterone is believed to be related to sex drive. It would be logical to expect men to be more highly sexed than women since they possess so much more of the stuff whizzing round their endocrine systems. However, this doesn't seem to be the case. Some men and women are highly sexed, some are lowly sexed and most of us are somewhere in between.

Inside the body, testosterone fuses with another substance called hormone-binding globulin. This effectively prevents large amounts of testosterone from being able to affect sex drive. It just might be the impact and vagaries of this process that are responsible for the differences within the sexes and between the sexes.

What's more, although testosterone therapy can replace sex drive in both men and women, it doesn't always do so. To complicate matters further, men who have been castrated, ie, have had their supply of testosterone removed, can experience both sexual desire and potency for up to thirty years after the castration. However, there is one group of women in the US who firmly believes in the strengthening capacity of testosterone. Calling themselves The Third Sex they masculinise themselves by taking regular high doses of androgen. Their characteristics are increased aggression, greater energy and greater drive (of all sorts), plus masculinisation of appearance and a great tennis serve.

BEHAVIOUR

Apart from being interesting to read about, why should any of these sex differences matter to us? The answer lies in the resulting behaviour. Although the number of actually proven sex differences is numerically small, they do exist. And it is on this variance that the survival of partnerships depends. It is the basis of our attraction. If sex difference didn't exist, we would be driven to invent it.

TRANSSEXUAL SEX

Male-to-female transsexuals report that, after the operation, the nerves in the pubic area often retain sensitivity and provide enough sensation to allow sexual activity to continue satisfactorily.

2

THE *physical* WOMAN

When you set eyes on an attractive woman for the first time, you see her outer self. You are looking at the 'external woman'. But beneath the surface, under that interesting skin, is a complex of identity-buffeting hormones and neurones that affect how she will project herself to any potential partner, including you. *So, don't mistake external appearances for reality.*

GETTING UNDER HER SKIN

If you were to visualise yourself making a journey of exploration through your lover's body, you'd be surprised how many of the sexual signals a woman sends and receives are mediated hormonally. It is these hormones that control.

1 **sexual drive,** how she comes on to you
2 **sexual desire,** how she responds
3 **sexual response,** consisting of **arousal and orgasm**

To complicate matters her special blend of hormones fluctuates. It changes in tune with her menstrual cycle, with pregnancy, breastfeeding and rate of recovery from childbirth. And every time the hormone blend re-mixes, her emotions go through a corresponding evolution. In addition, human identity is not always worn obviously. Often, a woman may look happy or sad but this is just the surface situation. Outward smiles and frowns often conceal contrasting inward states.

The exciting consequence is that you can forever be discovering new layers to the same woman. She is complex, multi-dimensional and a little like the weather in Britain – always in change. But she *is* exciting.

1. HER SEXUAL DRIVE

The first reason why she responds to your maleness is that she is driven by her hormones. The second, evolutionists would say, is her need to pass on her genes as widely as possible to ensure survival of her line. We've never been quite sure about that last since it doesn't seem to take the boon of birth control into account. The third is her drive to find a personal *meaning in life*.

In this third regard, sex undoubtedly provides a unique opportunity of learning about other people and ourselves. As a species, we are driven by curiosity. Sexually, we want to know this creature of the opposite gender. We want to delve down deep inside her and connect to the very essence of her being and we want to do so erotically.

A bit over the top for men? Laid on with a trowel? Well, think about it from your own perspective. In penetrating your partner you are actually, physically, moving as far inside her as you can. Short of surgery, you are trying to get so close you could be journeying into the centre of her being. Maybe, unconsciously, in our own sensual way, we are trying to get back to the Eden of pre-birth – a time of complete sensual containment when every particle of our skin was touched by a warm living sensual mother and where there were no outside elements to harm or distract us. Sexuality as a means to recapture an experience of earliest life?

Of course we don't consciously attempt this – or recall it. We are unable to do so since we have no words to describe the experience and psychologists now believe that clear memory only forms with speech. The impression *may* be buried inside us waiting to be brought out but *if* this is a sensual memory it inevitably takes a sensual closeness to evoke it.

So what – perhaps – we do in the act of sex is try, in our own unconscious way, to learn more about ourselves, our beginnings and what made us. Men and women each want to possess and be possessed, striving to assuage a deeply personal sense of artificial separateness.

2. HER SEXUAL DESIRE

What is it that *physically* creates sex drive? As we have said, **hormones**. Women possess some complicated ones – so mysterious that their role is not fully understood. The hormone that governs whether or not a woman puts out that extra little spark to make her irresistible is testosterone – or at least we think it is. Sex researchers now increasingly suspect that **testosterone** is responsible for four things – genital growth and sensitivity in women plus initial interest in sex **plus the drive to seek partners.** Women known to have high (free-ranging) testosterone levels usually also have high sex drive.

The **menstrual cycle** also plays its own part in how sexy a woman feels. There are times of the month when she may positively beat down the door to the bedroom and other times when she would far rather hibernate with a good book and a box of chocolates. If you graduate to any kind of a regular relationship, you would be advised to keep a chart for a couple of months so that you can get to recognise her high arousal peaks! Some women incidentally keep their own menstrual diary where they note down, not just physical symptoms but emotional ones too. These make for some enlightening reading.

In general most women feel very sexy 1) immediately before a period 2) sometimes during a period and 3) immediately after a period. Although there are a few women who 4) feel sexy in the middle of the month (during ovulation), many more don't. In general, the centre of the menstrual month is a fallow period for sexual desire. For a real dynamite experience focus on the night immediately *before* the period commences.

HOW TO KEEP A SEX DIARY

Start with Day 1 as the first day of your partner's period – the beginning of her new cycle. Note her mood, physical symptoms, signs of clumsiness or dexterity and her sexual response. Continue to do this faithfully for the whole of her menstrual month. Repeat the note-taking a second and third time. This should be enough to perceive any emotional or sexual patterns running throughout the month.

Sex diaries can also be a revelation for the woman involved. Here's what one woman wrote: "I feel sexy much less often than I realised. It wasn't till I saw it noted in black and white that this became clear. But I also realised there were certain times when my body just took off sexually. When we'd identified those we made the most of them, believe me. The amazing sex we had at these highly sensual periods more than made up for the lessened amount."

In addition, there is a lot of psychological research that shows both men and women become sexually aroused if previously they have experienced some other 'parallel' arousal, be it fear, anxiety or even anger. These emotions are again mediated by the hormones. *Shortly before the onset of menstruation* women are often on edge, emotionally bad-tempered and therefore physically aroused!

What about women who no longer have periods? Quite a few of them continue to experience fluctuating moods as if they were still menstruating, although this evens out in the fullness of time. Eventually, the essentials of good sex remain much the same – only without the fluctuations. It may take longer for arousal to happen, but from surveys of older women most reveal that they enjoyed sex as much, or even more, than before.

3. HER SEXUAL RESPONSE

You are also well aware that making love with the hands, tongue and whole body is important to a woman's good experience of sex. You even know that some women are capable of having more than one orgasm at a time. And with the possible exception of men from Mars, most ambitious lovers really do understand that 'slam bam, thank you M'am' is no longer acceptable.

But do you know exactly what takes place during her sexual response? Perhaps you assume that the same thing happens to her as happens to you? And that is never a wise thing to do when it comes to matters of explosively exciting sex where you want to make an impact of such cataclysmic proportion that she never looks at A.N.Other again.

LABIAL ERECTION

Let's assume that you've moved on to the sex act itself. The latest information from the US has now demonstrated that women get erections in a similar way to men. We now know, thanks to research into a possible Viagra Pill for women, that the area around the top of the labia, taking in the clitoris and extending down each side of the vaginal lips towards the perineum, contains spongy tissue. This fills up with blood and swells, in exactly the same way that the penis does. What makes it swell and become sexually sensitive are not quite the same things that affect men. And this is an important difference. If you assume that what works for you will automatically work for her, you are mistaken. If a woman finds herself being penetrated before she becomes aroused (literally before she gets her erection) she experiences the equivalent of you trying to stuff your flaccid penis inside her and perform gloriously with that.

AROUSAL

So what gets the female erection going? Where does a woman differ from her male lover? Three-quarters of women don't get turned on visually in the same way that most men do. Women rely more on suggestion, hence the powerful need for romance; female fantasies are much more poetic and low key (however, they still work!); and above all women rely on foreplay. This hideous word is a short cut description of the stroking, caressing, skin to skin contact, playing, and all-over body stimulation that most women adore. Quite a lot of men rate it highly too!

During the latter part of the arousal process many of the body muscles become tense. It's important to emphasise this because there's been a myth that says for a woman to enjoy sex she needs to relax. Her brain certainly needs to feel relaxed *mentally*, to trust, to be anxiety-free but her body actually responds in an opposite manner. Indeed, some women are so skilful at tensing their own body and in particular their genitals that they can bring themselves off to climax without any genital touching at all.

At the height of the arousal phase seventy-five per cent of women develop a 'sex flush'. This is a temporary strawberry-type rash that spreads rapidly from under the rib cage and all over the breasts.

THE CLITORIS

At the same time, just prior to orgasm, a tricky thing happens to the clitoris. This versatile little organ, which naturally you have been stroking and sucking and twirling delicately, disconcertingly retracts and becomes suddenly difficult to find. This can be disastrous because, if all that amazing attention you have been paying it suddenly ceases, the woman's arousal drains away. Women need continuous unbroken stimulation for them to be able to climax and in this very particular way *they differ radically from men*. Where men reach a point of inevitability, women don't. *Even when they are actually climaxing, experiencing the throes of ecstasy, once you stop the stimulation you stop the orgasm.* This is one reason why some women sometimes feel incomplete, even though they have experienced a climax. It's also the reason why many women don't experience multiple orgasm when they possess the potential. So hang on in there even if the effort is killing you.

MULTIPLE ORGASM

And what about multiple orgasm? These are of several different kinds. There's the sort where your partner has a series of small shallow orgasms. There's another where she experiences quite major climaxes, although divided by short intervals; there's a further sort where she may have a second, some five or ten minutes after the first; and there's a rare kind, identified by famous sex researchers Masters and Johnson in their laboratories, as 'status orgasmus'. This last consists of rapidly recurrent orgasms that are experienced as an intensely long drawn-out climax. There are probably dozens more but no Casanova of the sex age has yet started collecting them. They could form the basis for an interesting PhD.

ORGASM

Orgasm itself, even without its multiple option, remains varied. Singleton female orgasms can be long and strong, or short and weak Some women experience them around the clitoral area, some inside the vagina, some identify uterine contractions, particularly during pregnancy when they are easier to spot, some have G-spot climaxes that include a type of ejaculation and some women experience all over body climaxes where every inch of their frame shakes and vibrates. What's more, many of these variants can be experienced by one woman during her sexual lifetime.

If you're a strictly intercourse man you may be feeling dismayed by our constant return to the desirability of manual or oral stimulation of the clitoris. Perhaps you have been lucky enough to meet with one of the only 30 per cent of females who experiences orgasm through intercourse or G-spot sensation alone. Yes, it is possible. Research has demonstrated that the pull exerted by the to and fro of intercourse on the labia means that the labia creates a gentle but regular friction over the clitoris and this may be enough eventually to trigger climax. Great when it happens. But if you consider that at least 82 per cent of women are capable of experiencing climax but only 30 per cent of them actually do so without the aid of more direct clitoral stimulation, the odds are you'll need more than your faithful penis.

THE MYTH OF SIMULTANEOUS ORGASM

Incidentally, just in case you are still subscribing to the myth that the only true sexual experience is one of simultaneous orgasm, forget it. This is a dinosaur belief, best condemned to the tar pits. Just about any and every way to experience orgasm is a good one. And though some people swear by coming off together, others insist that concentrating so hard on timing detracts from full sensual enjoyment. Each to his own!

THE *female* PSYCHE

3

Because this is a book for men, we've started with the sex bits first. From a female point of view, we've begun in the wrong place. If we did this on a first date we'd be roundly rejected. What needs to precede sex is a *system of relating*.

For large chunks of the 20th century the 'system of relating' was fixed. Men made the moves; women encouraged and accepted them. Men were active socially and sexually; women were more passive. Times and systems change and the last 25 years have seen a revolution. Today's young women think it perfectly OK to take the initiative. If they want to have sex in casual circumstances they see no reason on earth why they shouldn't. (It is what men have always done, after all). Nor does the option of casual sex mean that long drawn-out passionate sex in an exclusive relationship is devalued. The change is that this is now seen as one of *several* options. Today's young women don't make such a big deal out of intercourse.

This means that sex has many different meanings for different times and occasions. The one common denominator is that every woman wants to think that you are interested in her as a human being, as a person, even if she is a stranger. *What she won't be keen on is to be viewed as a receptacle.*

This means that:
- ❦ the quickie
- ❦ the long drawn out games-playing occasion
- ❦ the friendship connection
- ❦ the sex on the cushions in the bedroom at the party occasion
- ❦ the revenge fuck
- ❦ tender love-making and
- ❦ passionate fusing of minds and bodies

. . . all have their place and all serve a particular dynamic. *Just so long as you believe she is a human being and treat her with respect.* (Lose sight of this and you're a dead duck). Expect to pursue and be pursued. In the 21st century, your woman is likely to come on to you. She may make more of the running; she may dictate what goes on in the bedroom. The new century finds this ordinary everyday behaviour. And it has its advantages. It means that you don't always have the onerous responsibility of making the play. It's really nice to discover someone fancies the socks off you. Just as long as you keep it firmly in mind that these are ordinary young women, making ordinary moves, who continue to be worth your respect.

There is emotional fall-out from such behaviour, however, and some women need to be kept firmly in touch with the concept of personal responsibility – yours and hers. If, for example, she seduces you, knowing you are married, she also knows (even if she tidies such information firmly to the back of her mind) that she cannot get your undivided attention. And if she doesn't seem to have taken this in, you owe it to her and to yourself to remind her every so often. The boot is on the other foot however if you seduce a married woman. Expect to feel pain when she can't meet with you at the weekends.

'Each to his own' or 'the selfish seduction' is a consumer ideology that leaves many casualties along the way. Women and men who treat relationships like jobs, only have an eye to the main chance and a belief that the

THE FEMALE SEXUAL BILL OF RIGHTS

Women in the 21st century believe that they have the right to:

- ❦ Get good sex
- ❦ Give good sex
- ❦ Be open about sex
- ❦ Sexually explore people and situations
- ❦ Pursue any man, regardless of his marital status

future will take care of itself. This consumer approach is rooted in a traditionally male pattern of relating that today's women are colonising and adapting. Thirty years ago, men expected to be able to set the pace in a sexual relationship, to dictate the shape and direction it took. Today, that pace and direction are up for grabs. It's not yet settled down as an entirely comfortable new dating system. But it's in the process of evolution.

THE ROMANTIC IDEAL

The shift in sexual lifestyles pivots on the fact that women are no longer willing to have an old-fashioned idea of feminine behaviour projected upon them. They don't expect to be little women at home – they expect to be equal partners. If you fall back on old patterns of expectation when you first meet your 'new' woman you'll be dooming the relationship before it even starts. Women have moved on. Women are voting not to make committed relationships with their feet. There are more single households and more women statistically unlikely to become mothers than ever before. Your attitude to women counts therefore, right from the first date.

So what kind of a paragon is it that the discerning woman might be attracted to? One woman described 'a man with the earning power of a banker, the empathy skills of a psychologist, the intellect of an academic, the body of a gymnast and Woody Allen's jokes'. Yet, by doing so, she's also projected an ideal – a contemporary one. Of course, we all do it. But the reality is that nobody can be ideal. Nobody is perfect, especially Woody Allen. Everyone displays down sides as well as up sides. Love doesn't guarantee happiness nor does good behaviour secure a partner's fidelity.

The obvious way for any man and woman to relate is to approach each other as brand new human beings with no preconceptions. Beginning from scratch, the task must be to discover exactly what the other person consists of; what kind of a character lives underneath the surface. Of course this has *always* been the obvious way but puzzlingly hasn't prevented men in the past from falling into any number of cunning traps.

SHED YOUR PRECONCEPTIONS

There's the cunning trap of outer appearance. We expect things from a woman from the moment we first see her. We get ideas about what we think she's like from the way her features are shaped, the manner in which she wears her clothes, the styles she chooses. And these are pictures we relate to because

🐛 We have known others like her
🐛 She unconsciously reminds us of a member of the family
🐛 We have seen similar images of people in the public eye

It's normal, it's natural – we can't help making associations from one person to another. So, we start off with preconceptions that may be completely erroneous. About the only way to get a real feel of an 'inner' or 'essential' individual these days is through the Internet where you can't actually hear or see her, only communicate directly to her imagination and writing skills.

So almost immediately we believe that we know things about a stranger and we project our beliefs on to her. The same goes for sexuality. Most men looking at Janna assumed that she was amazing in bed – they expected that her imagined confidence would allow her to be wild and experimental. The truth was that she was quiet and inhibited and because men had such unreal expectations, through no fault of her own, she tended to be disappointing.

If this is true of the women you fancy, spare a thought for yourself. How much of the true 'you' do you allow to appear? Are you confident enough to be open about inadequacy? Do you project a real picture of yourself onto others? Or do you project the person you would like to be?

CASE HISTORY

Janna was an exceptionally beautiful young woman whom most people would assume, on meeting her for the first time, would be supremely confident and able to pick any man she wanted. They could be forgiven for thinking that Janna was probably a top model, with a major income, an exciting social life and a zillion friends. These are the kind of assumptions we all make based on preconceptions of the lifestyle that some exceptionally beautiful young women lead. The clue to Janna's real personality lay in her eyes. If you looked carefully, hers were the eyes of a wild animal, wary and angry. For Janna was depressed, irrationally furious with her parents, able to hold down only the most menial of jobs as a shop assistant, regularly exploited by men who loved her and left her. She eventually had a serious breakdown.

There's a school of psychology that believes we learn and gain in tricky situations by acting 'as if'. If we behave 'as if' we are confident, we are more likely to get a date. Because we have actually got the date, our confidence increases. Next time we ask for a date we will feel more confident and the chance of acceptance increases. Building confidence in this way is an upward spiral based on acting 'as if'. Try it.

FEAR OR AGGRESSION?

One psychological study showed that women reacted to a threat with fear. By contrast, men reacted to the same threat with aggression. This may not be relevant to all men and women but it always pays to put the object of your desire at her ease.

Don't we *all* try to give the appearance of the person we would really like to be? Yet the problem is that we may find ourselves in deeper waters (sexually) than anticipated. One safeguard is to develop greater skills of empathy to anticipate a partner's anxieties and hidden hesitations.

FAMILY PSYCHOLOGY

There's the cunning trap of family psychology. Although we usually discuss our families and share information about where family members live, what they do and what they are like as individuals, we never discuss what kind of sexual example they may have given us. This is probably because it has never dawned on us that our own attitudes towards the expression of love, the ability to be warm and tactile, the confidence to let go sexually and to trust will have its foundations in what we have seen (or sensed) in our original family home.

Sex therapists often come up against problems caused in childhood by poor family examples. For example, women attending a group in order to learn how to climax, shared several common denominators. They had parents who:

- were unloving towards each other,
- never touched or cuddled
- were chronically inhibited on the subject of sex and who passed their inhibition, almost amounting to a phobia to their daughters.

From the outside these women looked like any other. So, if you meet a friendly, attractive female (and you have had a warm, loving family life yourself,) don't assume that this new friend comes from a similar background. She may not.

We also, unconsciously, look for points of familiarity in a new partner. The person we feel most at home with, most comfortable with, may remind us, without our knowing it, of a parent or brother or sister. It is easy then to slip into family patterns of relating which is fine if the new partner really does behave as you anticipate. But, if your girlfriend surprises you by coming from a very different culture, some of your assumptions that feel perfectly normal to you may turn out to be completely unacceptable to her.

CASE HISTORY

Paolo came from a large family where tempers flared quickly, shouting matches were common but cooled just as rapidly and were forgotten in a minute. Marie came from a family that considered the display of anger to be sinful. If you were angry you were effectively attacking the world you lived in. Marie not unnaturally found it extremely difficult to be swept into sexual activity with Paolo immediately after a row. Paolo found the shouting normal and arousing, Marie saw the shouting as pathological and fearful. The two family cultures came into serious conflict and it was only through the intervention of counselling that the couple learned what had actually gone wrong.

LOSING FACE WITH FRIENDS AND MATES

There's also the cunning trap of expectations that are formed by what we think the *outside world* expects of us. If you live in Los Angeles for example, you must have a fast car, expensive clothes, a thin hard body, perfect features or enough cash for remedial plastic surgery. You are nothing and no-one if you don't seem glamorous. This extends to choice of mates. If you turn up with someone less than beautiful on your arm, you don't feel good because you suspect that your friends are adversely rating you. This also extends to what happens sexually between the two of you. It is assumed that you will both be sexually sophisticated – willing for anything. God help you if you aren't. Back in Europe, some of this 'willing for anything" expectation is snaking its way into sexual attitudes. It's insidious and devious. There's a sense that if you are *not* willing to do anything, you not only let a partner down, you believe there is something wrong with you. Yet common sense tells us this is nonsense.

If you come from a fundamentally religious background, the opposite sexual assumption will be prevalent. This can be damaging in a

---

THE PRELIMINARY SIX-POINT PLAN

1 Take your time. Don't be so compelled by your sex drive that you frighten her off on the first date.

2 Find out about her – her background, what she's like and what she likes.

3 Use 'warmth' moves once you feel she's interested. Touch her on the elbow, help her when crossing the road, use excuses for informal touch. If you're strolling together hold her hand or tuck it under your arm. Timing is an issue. If you do this from day one you will be too quick off the mark. Judge the pace.

4 Be open to her, listen to what she says and show that you are responding by nodding or making little comments. If you dominate the conversation (occasionally a masculine trait) smack yourself firmly on the hand, bite your lips and focus on her instead.

5 Women like men from whom they think they can learn. If you don't feel particularly knowledgeable, bone up on things that interest her – anything from psychology to horticulture.

6 Cultivate your sense of humour – it's sexy, and the whole point of making love is that it should be fun.

---

different way. One young woman, the daughter of an ardent Presbyterian – a much older father – had been so terrorised into not displaying a jot of sexuality that when it came to the permitted circumstance, ie. marriage, she found it completely impossible to let go her tight control. A strict religious upbringing, where sex is associated with hellfire and deep sin, is a common denominator for women with orgasmic problems.

With this number of hidden obstacles it's a wonder that anyone's love life ever takes off. But we manage, we do the utmost we can, we struggle instinctively to love and encourage. Now using this book, we want to help you create the most favourable circumstances in which a love affair can take root.

HEIGHTEN THE EMOTIONS

Communicate *verbally*: one excellent method of getting on your partner's wavelength is to ask her for a sexual biography. She likes it and *you* get clued up. Think back to the earliest days.

- What example of sensuality did her parents set? Were they physically affectionate? To each other? To her?
- What was her parents' attitude towards sex? What might she have learned from them?
- When did she first discover sex? With other people? With herself?
- How did early sexual relationships influence her? Were these good or bad experiences? Does she think they may have influenced her choice of subsequent partners?

As you ask questions, disclose information about yourself in return. Compare notes. See if there are areas in your separate histories that match. Talk about the differences. One of the results of living in a culture where discussion about sex is still partly foreign is that we don't normally collect such information. Yet by sharing the answers we work out what is going to encourage each of us in a new relationship to find trust and be turned on.

Use *warmth moves* with each other.
- Sometimes look longer than usual into your partner's eyes.
- Turn towards the other more than you would do normally.

- Smile more than usual.
- Make small touching movements. For example, when standing together, stand behind your partner, cuddling lightly against her body, with both arms around the waist; put an arm around your partner; caress and massage your partner's back.
- Brush your partner's hair sensuously – it feels wonderfully intimate

HEIGHTEN THE PHYSICAL SENSATION

As the relationship progresses from talking to touch, don't be in a tearing hurry to initiate full intercourse. Go for touch techniques – use the wonderful arts of sensual massage. You might begin with:

- Maximising the erotic potential of the foot. A foot massage can be incredibly sexy – vary firmer pressures (to relieve tired feet) with teasing, sensual strokes.
- Unashamedly, go for a full body massage, rather than just sex. Touch is probably the most important and enhancing aspect of any relationship. The skin is the body's second most sensual organ after the brain. Use circling strokes, warm hands, warmed massage oil and a warm room. Start pressing with the full hand, always stroking away from the spine and always *slowly*. When you've covered the body thoroughly with a firm touch, deliberately lighten up using fingertips only. Make a final third round, using the finger*nails*.
- Treat the genitals to a massage in much the same way as you would the rest of the body. Don't aim at climax and *make it clear to your partner this is not the focus*. Follow up a body massage by using the same circling techniques on the genitals, only with smaller, more sensitive circling strokes and methodically cover the entire area from inner thighs upwards, culminating at the clitoris. Don't do a genital massage *unless* you have covered the rest of the body first. It won't have anything like the same impact.

Don't turn this into intercourse towards the end of the evening. By giving her a foretaste of sensuality and by leaving her aroused but unpenetrated, she will urgently want to snuggle extremely close indeed at the next meeting. What you are doing here is building up her erotic feeling; teaching her to associate you with an extreme of sensuality.

*t*he EMOTIONAL WOMAN

4

It's said that some men don't acknowledge the brain as the largest sex organ. Yet the human brain not only sends out commands to the rest of the body, it ensures that the skin feels aroused and organises all the sensations that turn desire into response. Women's brains work sexually just like men's *except* that women don't single out good looks. Women tend to respond more to someone's overall impact than their prettiest feature. The more personal the better. Put an interesting idea into a woman's head and she will get turned on. The 'internal' woman, the one that sizes you up and assesses your appeal is just as important as the 'external woman', the one who may physically react.

A vital part of her response system has been put in place not by you but by the people she has known from the very start of life. Your woman is part baby, part little girl. She's the rowdy teenager and the thoughtful 20 year old. All these in addition to her present self. On this backlog of love and conditioning rests the success or failure of your pursuit. If her mind, influenced by history, decides that you don't suit her, it doesn't matter how skilfully you carry out the butterfly flick – you won't get her. So, finding out what appeals to her brain is an absolute priority.

IMPACT OF YOUR SCENT ON HER BRAIN

Some of what will work is a lottery. If you smell wrong, she will instinctively withdraw although instinctively may not be the correct word since actually her brain has made a rapid assessment of your body odour, enabling her to make a quick decision. Even body scent can be partially altered if you change your diet, but I doubt that many any of us can be bothered to go to such extremes. Similarly, if, through no fault of your own, you strongly remind her of someone she has disliked in the past, she may endow you with his characteristics and be unable to appreciate your particular charms.

If, however, the signs augur well, and she perceives no reasons for rapid withdrawal, there are very specific ways in which you might conduct the beginning (indeed the entirety) of the relationship to optimise your chances of success. Please understand, when we are talking success here, we are not discussing notches-in-the-belt seduction. We are talking about the setting-up-of-a-first-class-sexual-friendship that will, with any luck, transform into greater total love.

HER NEED FOR YOUR HONESTY

While, ideally, most women want romance and the possibility of commitment, they want it on truthful terms. Women certainly don't want men's pretence. The best sex, many women believe, is orchestrated between people who trust each other, can talk about anything and can joyfully explore each other's differences. If, therefore, you think there is a remote chance of wanting a special woman long-term, be prepared to tune into these emotional requirements and then cherish them.

YOUR NEED FOR YOUR HONESTY

The trouble with seduction is that it reeks of manipulation. In the short term, for the object of your desire, it may be wonderful to be on the receiving end. It may also feel like a personal triumph to you, the seducer. But if you know that someone has responded to actions not representative of your true self and *it is important that you feel loved for your true self*, then you will never feel properly loved or accepted by seduction alone. If, on the other hand, you are strong enough and daring enough to reveal yourself, complexes and all, your loving and

'I' AND 'YOU'

There is a verbal communication method that helps overcome the blunt and blatant impact of words that are unwelcome. Most people, when complaining, automatically say 'you'. 'You keep getting this wrong.' 'You keep missing the spot.' 'You are failing to give me a climax.'

Try getting someone to say these to your face and see how you feel. Our guess is that your reaction won't be positive for the excellent reason that using 'you' all the time is accusatory. It is as if your partner is pointing a finger at you and saying 'it's all your fault". They may not intend it like that. But that is how the meaning comes out.

Under these conditions, a partner's reaction is first and foremost not to co-operate, but to defend. And when people are defensive they don't usually feel like crawling back into bed and giving you an amazing time.

An alternative way of dealing with a difficult issue is to come from 'I'. 'I feel unhappy because we are not seeing much of each other.' 'I love it when you stroke my nipples.' 'I feel really uncomfortable when my stomach is massaged. I have an over-sensitive stomach'

Coming from 'I' means that you take the responsibility for the problem, that this is your problem, not your partner's but that she might possess the power to help. The usual response to this more subtle approach is sympathy and a desire to help. By opening up in this way that you are going to draw your mate much closer.

your sexuality stand a better chance of evolving into something very special. And of course the same goes for her.

Honesty between two people demands at least two different kinds of strength. The first is the strength to talk truthfully. The second is the ability to deal with the truth when it arrives. It's easier to conceal, it's easier to stick with half-truths and, very occasionally there are times when this may be truly appropriate. But increasingly we believe that the best route of all is to open up about yourself. Some people manage this better than others and that is because there are skills to the way honesty can be handled.

OPENING UP

Most of us know that opening up (who we are, what we like and what has gone on in our past) is an integral part of a new relationship. Opening up is important because the information you offer gives the other person something to relate to. Your lively words allow her to respond, to talk back, to compare notes, to contribute her own personal stories in exchange. If we remain silent, we not only give her little or nothing to work on but we also give the impression that we are withholding, sitting back, judging and probably judging negatively. This is extremely uncomfortable. So it is vital to offer snippets of information.

LISTENING

It is also vital not to hog the conversation, never allowing the other person to contribute. If she is shy or slow about herself, ask her about herself. Encourage her to tell you about her background, where she comes from, what she does. In order to gain confidence and to open up she needs to feel that you are interested. And in order to believe that, she needs to actually see you listening to her. There are few things more annoying than someone who asks you a question but who then checks out the whole of the rest of the room, does not respond and has no idea of what you've said when you finish.

All these listening skills should be used in bed while lying close together, preferably in each other's arms. If she can't see your face because of the way you are lying you can still nod so that she feels the nod, still murmur replies and also indicate, through hugs and caresses that you are responsive to any suggestions. If the conversation is an unhappy one and she is upset, you can use this comforting body touch to reassure her while she's speaking.

LISTENING SKILLS

You might:

- Nod your head to indicate that you're taking in her words

- Say 'um' and 'yes' and 'I see' etc to show that you are following the flow

- Keep your gaze on her face – don't turn away, walk around the room or display your back

- Don't do something else while she's talking.

- Respond, verbally, once she has finished, in such a way that you show you have really heard what she's said and try to incorporate her comments in your following remark. A good conversation builds up brick by brick; a bad one demolishes the other person's position.

first MOVES

5

First occasions of love-making are sometimes nerve-wracking. At least one of you is usually anxious about the way things will go. Often there will be small problems that you need to negotiate. The listening skills come in useful here. So too does the 'I' not 'you' exercise.

What can you expect in the way of first night nerves? Sally explained that she had very different reactions to first sex depending on what stage of life she had reached. 'When I was a teenager, although 'going all the way' was a big deal, I'm not sure I thought much about it. I was so keen to get it together with this boy and it all happened so spontaneously that we just did it. I think I was lucky in that sex went very well from the start and that we had spent a while getting to know each other beforehand, including a lot of very passionate necking.

'This first relationship split up after three years and after that I experienced some anxieties. My confidence had been knocked. I would freeze and feel nothing. And it wasn't till I met someone who bothered to give me some reassurance and some getting-to-know-each-other time before we went to bed that I could respond again. Much later in life, after my marriage split up, I met a new man by whom I was very intrigued but I was also very nervous. He spent hours over me, just stroking and playing. In fact, we reached a stage where I thought we weren't going to have intercourse because we'd been fooling around like little kids for such a long time. And we didn't – have intercourse. Which is why, the *next* time we got together, I was really, really enthusiastic. And it was wonderful.'

Sally told us that her first time reactions were directly connected to how good she felt about herself at the time. Bearing this in mind, it makes sense to do some tuning-in with a new friend, in order to find out where she is in her love life. If there is any reason to think that she is going to be nervous, take your time. But don't just talk about the situation, stroke, caress, kiss her passionately, tell her intimate tales, move your hands around her body and encourage her to do the same to you. Women find a man who holds back from intercourse extremely attractive. But women also like warmth and sensuality. So stroke while you talk. The longer there is a build up of sensual activity, the better love-making gradually becomes. If you think of sexuality as a form of energy, humming and speeding through the body, you realise it makes sense to generate huge amounts of it on the theory that a massive build-up results in a seismic explosion.

CHECKING OUT HER NERVES

Assessing your woman's anxieties therefore is important since your timing will affect how well the first attempts go. If, for example, you instantly demand sex from her she will think of you as a pushy person and may well resist.

- Think about your behaviour.
- If you identify yourself as being in one hell of a hurry, are you actually pushy?
- Or are you very needy?
- Or are you driven by sexual desire?

None of these situations have much to do with her, do they? Even the sexual desire. You may argue that sexual desire is provoked by her but

FIRST TIMERS

Tilly's first sexual experiences were with another sixth former in the school library. 'We'd made love in practically every way you can think of, barring intercourse. Of course, it was terribly exciting because of the risk of being caught. Amazingly, we never were. Eventually, we knew we would have intercourse. We were very responsible. I got myself put on the Pill, we waited till it would take effect and then stayed the night at a friend's house. First intercourse was all right. But after the incredible stimulation we'd given each other in the library, it came as a bit of a disappointment. It took the next couple of months, to work out how to combine foreplay with intercourse. After that, it got much better.'

in fact it is only triggered by her – it is actually provoked by *you*, inside your head. And what is inside your head should not be thrust upon someone when they are not ready for it.

So just how can you check out the state of play with regards her love life, her self- confidence and what she may want from a new partner, that is, you? In the previous chapter we talked about her family, what kind of people they are, how they relate to each other and what example of warmth and loving they have offered their children. Hopefully you will have revealed similar information about yourself to her. Here we offer suggestions for a revealing conversation about sexual experience.

A SEXUAL CONVERSATION

Now that things are getting more physical this is the time to move on to a more sensual version of each other's lives. You might exchange information on:

- First sexual feelings
- First partners of the opposite sex
- First sexual exchanges. Did you/she go all the way? Or was there a long run-in? What were the first experiences like?
- Self-stimulation. Does/did she/you do this? If so, when did it start? What were the first experiences like? How did it match up to later sexual experience?
- The first important relationships. What were they like? What kind of a person was the first partner? How did sex go with them?
- The next important relationships. How have these affected you/her? Where do they leave the pair of you now with regards mood, expectations, emotional scars?

We are not suggesting you pin your woman against a wall and interrogate her in the glare of a bright light. Clearly anything as intimate as the suggested exchange needs to be done casually, while cuddling and making out. Lots of body reassurance, warmth moves and sensual touch should help her unwind.

REASSURANCE

- If she shows hesitation she needs more reassurance.

- If she is reluctant to disclose things about herself, set an example by going first.
- If she's shy, tell her 'It was like this for me. How was it for you?'
- Phrases such as 'I get the impression this is hard for you to talk about' sometimes work wonders.
- Or commiseration: 'Yes, when sex goes wrong it can be destroying, can't it.'
- Or praise: 'How well you told that difficult story'.
- Or reassurance: "I get the sense that life hasn't treated you very kindly for a while'.

DEALING WITH YOUR NERVES

So far we've talked as if you were an experienced counsellor with not a jot of doubt or hesitation in your ability to carry off such an intimate negotiation. Most of us are not such matchless operators, however. The thought of launching into such a profound exchange may seem:

- Intrusive
- Nerve-wracking
- Beyond your experience or capability

Intrusion: If, as you launch into your seemingly casual questions, you receive the distinct impression that you are intruding, pay attention to the feeling. You may be venturing into difficult territory too quickly and too soon. Take an emotional step backwards and wait a while. Provided the rest of things go well, don't be afraid to try again. If you repeatedly gain the impression of intrusion however you might use the following approach.

'I've been trying to ask you about yourself for some time now and I get the impression that this is difficult for you. Is there a problem here?'

'I see. Tell me more.'

Or: 'I don't want to be intrusive but I do want to get to know you better. Can you tell me something about your own life?'

Or even: 'I've told you quite a lot about my love life but I don't feel I'm hearing much from you. The trouble is, this is beginning to feel one-sided. Do me a favour, tell me a little'

STRENGTHENING YOUR CONFIDENCE

If apprehensive, there is a useful technique called **behavioural rehearsal**. This is where you picture, in your mind, the situation that you may shortly be facing. And it really helps at those moments when you don't know what to say.

Picture:

Scene 1. You are sitting next to your woman friend on the couch with your arm around her. She is leaning back against you and you have been listening to a CD. As you listen, you remark casually, 'I love that melody, it has really romantic connotations for me. Do you have any songs or numbers that bring back the memories?'

Say the words out loud. Imagine the woman next to you, listening to your comment as you murmur them into her ear. Try saying the same kind of thing out loud again, only making it different enough to clarify that you are asking her a question.

How did that feel? If you felt anxious while you were having an imaginary conversation, keep at it. It really helps to rehearse. If you were tense while saying your lines repeat them a third time. Keep repeating them until you are perfectly comfortable.

Picture:

Scene 2. Imagine that you are still on the couch with the woman friend but she has not yet answered you. You lean towards her and kiss her on the neck or on the side of the face. And then you let go and move back a bit. She looks at you but still doesn't speak.

You are puzzled. You look at her enquiringly and then say 'I don't want to be intrusive but I do want to get to know you better. I'd love to know more about you. Tell me a little.'

USING ASSERTION TECHNIQUE

Another helpful method to give you courage is that of assertion training. This works on the premise that the worst thing about tackling a difficult situation is taking the first step. And that the more you tackle successfully, the more confident you feel about yourself and the further you can go next time. For this particular situation therefore you might:

1 List six difficult moments in the relationship that you envisage

2 Label the list from one to six, with one for the easiest task, two for the next easiest and so on.

3 Starting with the easiest, try tackling the problems on the list and work your way down to the most difficult.

In this way, not only do you achieve change but you also create confidence. If something doesn't work, simply go back a step and wait till you feel better before attempting it again.

Again, go through the scene, saying your words out loud, rehearsing them over and over until you feel comfortable. What sort of a reaction do you think you might get? What are your worst fears? Do you fear rejection? Or do you simply not know how to handle things if she remains uncommunicative?

She is unlikely to reject you, since virtually everybody likes someone taking an interest. And she will almost certainly offer some answer. If she really can't say much, you can picture yourself giving her a big hug and saying 'I can see that you don't want to talk right now. But I'd love to hear a little about you some time.' And leave things at that.

The point of the rehearsal method is to let yourself say out loud what would be helpful when it comes to the real thing. And pretty obviously, you can go on to rehearse just about any scenario you think useful.

Beyond your experience or capability: If your instincts tell you that, by error, you have picked someone with major emotional problems or who is so seriously tricky you doubt your capacity to act as 'counsellor', then it's useful to recognise this. Don't be afraid of backing off a relationship if you feel sure it's not for you. This is the mature thing to do. If you fear that you are, in some way deserting this friend, you might, as tactfully as possible, point her in the direction of a real counsellor or therapist.

If going over the top is not
your style, practise a bit.
Useful phrases are:

I'm crazy about you.

You're a beautiful woman

*I am so turned on by your
body.*

*I am completely hooked by
your brain.*

I adore making love to you.

*You are a very sensual
woman.*

*You are becoming very
special to me.*

*I've thought about you
all day.*

*When I went home, I sat
down and wrote this
poem/letter to you.*

ENCOURAGEMENT

Earlier in this chapter we've talked about the best way to voice problems. Coming from 'I' and not 'you' is one good approach. But, if you are keen to improve your partner's lovemaking without her feeling criticised, always include something encouraging about her techniques alongside your request. For example: 'I adore the way you stroke my whole body. Your touch is marvellous. I'd love it if you'd stroke my penis in the same way as you do my stomach.'

However this is a book about improving your techniques for the benefit and ultimate enjoyment of the *woman* in your life. We believe that encouragement should be a key word for everyone, in every walk of life, especially in the bedroom. As sexual relationship therapists we are big on encouragement. Children learn faster through being encouraged. Workers work harder through feeling encouraged. And lovers feel happier if they think they are adored – an extreme form of encouragement! So let your woman know she is adored.

Of course, anything will do as long as it shows that your mind is erotically focused on her. We are not suggesting that you make any statement you don't mean. But many people find it surprisingly difficult to say how much they value their partner – somehow they expect this long-suffering individual to know by osmosis. We're reminded of the forthright phrase 'Of course I loves you, I fucks you, don't I?' It's a bad joke because no one knows they are loved unless they are verbally told so and unless the statement is regularly and repeatedly born out by caring, thoughtful behaviour it isn't true.

We learn how to be open and loving from our parents but, if we are unlucky enough to get parents who wouldn't dream of saying 'I love you, darling", we don't lay down the skills early enough in our brain patterns for this to happen spontaneously. *But the skills can be learned.* Try practising some passion in front of the mirror and feel the words while you are saying them. Use the rehearsal method.

'HEAVY PETTING'

We were fascinated to read recently that there are chemical reasons why two people become attached to each other. Apparently every time we have an orgasm we stimulate the production of the hormone oxytocin. Women produce oxytocin when they give birth and when they breast

HEAVY PETTING – HOW TO DO IT

1 Stroke your partner through her clothes.

2 Stroke your partner under her clothes.

3 Slipping off some of the clothes but not necessarily all, continue to stroke.

4 Stroke the top half of her body.

5 Graduate to the bottom half of her body.

6 Let your hands stray, as if by accident, across her genitals.

7 As you caress her inner thighs make sure that your fingers brush against her labia.

8 Let this 'accidental' brushing increase so that your hand is almost flickering across the genitals.

9 Pull her close to you and with slippery fingers, draw two of them up her genitals starting below the entrance to the vagina and ending on her pubic mound, making sure that they 'catch' on the clitoris on the way up. Do this a lot. There still needs to be a kind of accidental 'feel' about this even though, by now, both of you know that it is anything but. Lubrication is the secret of success here. If she is not wet enough, use her own juices or your saliva to make her so.

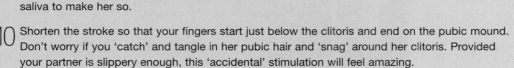

10 Shorten the stroke so that your fingers start just below the clitoris and end on the pubic mound. Don't worry if you 'catch' and tangle in her pubic hair and 'snag' around her clitoris. Provided your partner is slippery enough, this 'accidental' stimulation will feel amazing.

11 Assuming that she hasn't exploded into climax yet (and a lot of women will) shorten the stroke again so that you are brushing upwards on the clitoris alone.

CASE HISTORY

Fiona is a 49 year old woman who found herself comforted by an old friend shortly after her long-term relationship broke up. 'Everything about him happened comfortably. He kissed me as if he'd always known how. He slid his arms around me as though he'd done it for years. We kissed and hugged and groped and groaned like teenagers. It was marvellous.

'On about the third date we rolled all over my living-room floor just hugging and kissing and rubbing our bodies together through our clothes. But we didn't immediately take everything off and go to bed. Which suited me perfectly. I needed this time to get used to being sexual with someone new. In the end the invitation to stay the night came from me – not him. I was so intrigued by all this unpressured sex and the way in which it let me respond at my own pace, that it had the effect of totally turning me on. I just wanted to tear his clothes off and get into bed.

'And when we did, he gave me a massage in which he very cleverly allowed his fingers to brush against my clitoris and I practically erupted. I was so close to climax that I begged him to come inside me and he did, in spite of the fact he still had most of his clothes on. He was brilliant.'

feed and it is one of the ingredients that encourage bonding between mother and child. The theory also goes that the oxytocin stimulated during climax encourages us to bond to a lover more strongly.

One marvellous scenario that leads in to early love-making is 'heavy petting'. This is what men and women used to do in the pre-Pill days when, if you had intercourse, you probably also had a baby. 'Heavy petting' effectively allowed each of you to climax without taking the risk of penetration. We're not advocating that you persistently substitute this for the joys of sexual intercourse, but a subtle variation, carried out two or three times at the beginning of an intimate relationship may help you bond, and initiate trusting conversation.

Don't worry if she doesn't climax. This is just a finding out game but one that can be extraordinarily sensual. If you repeat and prolong the sequence the next time you get together, her response is likely to deepen. Provided the repetition of the stroke and the lubrication are adequate and assuming you become more knowledgeable and daring from session to session, she is highly likely to climax, if not on the first few occasions, then eventually. Should she appear to approach climax, but nevertheless doesn't tilt over into it, you might ask eventually, how you could vary the touch to make the stimulation more intense.

BODY WARMTH

The way we touch people makes an impression from the moment we meet. If we touch with warmth and reassurance, we invite warmth and appreciation in return. If we caress sensually, we provoke sensuality. Yet caressing does not spring spontaneously to everyone's hands. If we are hesitant over touch, that hesitancy communicates itself.

We first learn about touch at the hands of our parents. Skin to skin contact, cuddling and hugging are all early childhood experiences on which we build our later confidence and sexuality. Dr James Prescott, an American neuro-psychologist, claims that his work with primitive societies shows that people who are physically affectionate towards their children generally live in non-violent cultures. He writes that the positive benefits of warm affectionate touching during infancy may sometimes be undone by emotional repression in teenage. This can fortunately be mitigated provided there is a permitted degree of sensual pleasure from peers during adolescence.

Dr Prescott believes that a dose of sensuality in later life can socialise and introduce people to pleasure that they should have known earlier but didn't. Indeed, we know that touch can be used in an infinite number of ways. It can eliminate aggression, heal a quarrel, help deal with feelings of grief. Embracing a friend while you give bad news cushions the impact, stroking, patting and hugging your spouse, your children and your friends can let them know how much you care for them.

A television documentary made some years ago about touching showed that shoppers remembered the shop assistant better if she briefly touched them when she proffered their change. Research on job interviews shows that interviewers receive a more favourable impression of the applicant who shakes their hand than the one who does not. American research indicates that patients touched by their nurses were reassured, their anxiety reduced and they calmed down. Even patients in a coma registered a significant response when a nurse routinely took their pulse.

Close body contact at the early stages of a relationship, once you are past the getting-to know each other stage but before you have graduated to the full-body-sexual-intercourse stage, can lay the groundwork for a sensual, warm, expressive friendship.

SMALL TOUCH MOVES

There are a number of small ways in which we can learn to be more demonstrative. The following are just a few:

1 When you say hello to someone, shake their hand.

2 When you say goodbye, touch their arm.

3 If you are talking to a friend, make a point of touching them on the arm when emphasising something in the conversation.

4 When walking with a friend, put your arm through theirs for a while. Alternatively, and if appropriate, put an arm around their waist for a short time.

5 If you feel warm towards someone, give them a farewell hug.

6 Start kissing your friends hello and goodbye.

LARGER TOUCH MOVES

1 Stand up against her back and hug her tight into your body.

2 Dance, snuggled into each other's curves.

3 Lie, her back to your front, in the spoons position.

4 Sit her, facing you, across your knees, with your hands cupped to her buttocks to give her stability.

5 Stretch a long arm around her waist and rest the hand on hip, as far towards her pelvis as possible.

6 As you walk, put your arm round her waist but drop it to her buttocks as you move.

WATER GAMES

Water games people play can include:

- Washing each other's hair
- Scrubbing each other's backs in the bath
- Giving each other a foot bath and scrubbing each foot with peppermint (tingling) massage foam
- Giving each other a Thai soap-sud massage where you first anoint your beloved with a foam of bath suds and then slip and slide across her body with your own. *Not* advisable if you are heavy.

Our emphasis on taking things slowly and nurturing a woman's sense of wellbeing is above all designed to impress her 'internal' self. The sooner she feels flooded with warmth and trust towards you, the sooner she will want to fall on your body and make much of it. Keep cuddling.

6 falling IN LOVE

The sub-text of this book is how to make love to a woman – not just make sex. Love is an important word in female vocabulary and often gives women permission to be sexual in the first place. If they enjoy sex *without* being in love, many women believe there is something wrong with them. Women are also their own worst enemies. They judge themselves negatively for displaying the mildest of assertive sexual behaviour. Research on telephone usage has shown, for example, that while women believe they would be thought badly of by men for daring to grasp the receiver and ask a man out, men think this would be bliss. So love, as opposed to sex, is probably important to your partner.

Falling in love confers benefits. It can be marvellous, joyful, rewarding, life-enhancing, all-embracing, one of humanity's natural highs. The state of love possesses the ability to take you out of a dull routine by tingeing every simple action with a special quality. It makes life worthwhile – it gives purpose to existence. It's free, it's available to anyone regardless of age, economic status or class and it is the focus of entire industries woven around supplying songs, cards, books, gifts, meals, foods, music – all in the name of love. It can also kill you, but let's stick to the upside for the time being!

WHAT IS LOVE?

Poets and philosophers have been asking this question for centuries. Here's Anne's description of what love means to her : 'Idling away adoring hours under sunlit blue skies, being filled with warm, overflowing feelings for the man at whose side I'm lucky enough to walk; that's me in love. I leave one lover's side and fly rapidly to another. They're both marvellous and I care deeply for each but with totally different sets of feelings. But that's me in love – again. I look at my children and realise for the millionth time what utterly superior, adorable, well-bred, intelligent and attractive beings they are. I'm definitely in love with them. So that's me in love once more.

'Some people make me high with lunatic passion. Others have me contented to live for years at a low ebb of tenderness (but it's love, nevertheless). I've been jealous. I've been non-committal, caring mostly for men but deeply for one woman. I am able to love someone without ever having sex with him. I can work with someone until the working relationship reaches a stage of intimacy that's nigh on sexual. Or I can have a wonderful sexual relationship with a regular lover but spend little other time with him at all.

'These are all facets of me and my ability to love, and I'm not unique. But this is why, when asked to define what love is, most people boggle with the effort to constrain such a variety of feelings to a single word. One of the remarks critics make when I describe the happy variety of my loving feelings is: 'You can't really know what love is if you can't distinguish it.' What we feel they mean is that their own lives are so circumscribed that they have never allowed themselves the freedom of spirit to open up to more than one sensation of love.'

LOVE COMES IN THREE DIFFERENT VARIETIES

Throughout the world there are statisticians who research and codify these aspects of *la grande passion*. John Lee of Toronto University, for instance, has produced a typology of love. The three primary types of loving are, he found, fairly independent of each other. They consist of:

- 🐛 **Eros** (from the name of the Greek god of love)
  Characteristics: immediate physical attraction, sensuality, self-confidence, fascination with beauty, close intimacy and rapport with a partner.

- 🐛 **Ludus** (from the Latin for 'game')
  Characteristics: playfulness, focused on pleasure and free commitment

- 🐛 **Storge** (from a Greek word meaning 'natural affection')
  Characteristics: affection, companionable love and devoid of passion

It would of course be possible to feel each of these for different partners, or each of these in turn for one partner. During a relationship, loves goes through several stages.

LOVE COMPATIBILITY

Two 'storgic' lovers might expect to have the best chance of a lasting relationship while two 'ludic' lovers would have the least chance. 'Ludic' lovers would, however, have a lot more fun for as long as the affair endured.

Imagine some of the clashes, though, if the types intermix: a 'ludic' male may resent a 'storgic' female for trying to trap him into relationship, while she accuses him of playing games just to get her body; 'eros' may insist on making out immediately while 'storge' is most aroused by postponing sex.

LOVE'S ALTERATIONS

Whatever kinds of love you go for at different times in your life, US sociologist D.H. Knox has discovered that the more practical experience you get (e.g. in marriage) the more realistic you are likely to become about love. Perhaps this explains why we are never able to recreate the knockout feelings of that first love affair. Much as we want it again, a little inner voice points out all the inadequacies of powerful romance.

We are rarely warned that love may change. And love also sees with its own eyes, for lovers suffer from what Toronto University researchers Kenneth and Karen Dion call the 'distorting mirror' effect. Their research shows that lovers select inside their minds the way in which they *want* to see each other emotionally. What is more, they not only distort the perception of each other's appearance but they also become selective about their romantic memories. It's much easier to remember the happy, witty moments when your beloved told funny stories than the time she almost attacked you with a breadknife for eating the last cornflake.

THE VALUE OF LOVE

What is the value of this distortion by romantic love? One suggestion is that romantic feelings act as the supporting girders of a brand new love affair to keep it from toppling as it rises above the ground. The firmer the structure of love, the better you will feel about each other as you take risks and the greater the incentive becomes to stay together.

There's an old saying that opposites attract. They may indeed do so but their relationship doesn't make for the ideal marriage bond. Bentler and Newcomb of the University of California have deduced that a marriage is likely to last if you and your partner are similar in personality and if you are sensitive enough to realise your own shortcomings.

LOVE'S SMELLS

What is it that makes one person feel right and another feel wrong? According to Wilson and Nias, of the Institute of Psychiatry, London, the answer appears to be pheromones. Pheromones are substances that, when emitted as an odour by an animal, have the power to attract and stimulate a potential mate. Scientists have discovered a similar substance in humans. We are not generally conscious of being attracted to the body smells emitted by our sex partners, although we are aware when they smell bad! Nevertheless, many people are turned on by their partners' sweat; many men are aroused by the under-arm and vaginal odours of their women and many women are attracted by the male genital odours.

HOW TO MARRY A MILLIONAIRESS

'You can't help whom you fall in love with'. It's a useful argument but only partially accurate. Apparently, you can. The old-fashioned parents who used to send their daughters on world trips to get them away from undesirable lovers and meet up with a better class of person knew what they were doing. The love research proves that you are likely to meet and be attracted to someone in your immediate vicinity; and social circles and environments can often be controlled. If you want to marry a millionairess, go and move in wealthy circles!

Not all the young ladies exposed to the healing properties of a world-cruise manage to forget Mr Wrong. Absence *can* make the heart grow fonder and, said the late Professor Hans Eysenck, it's more likely to do so if you are an introvert (someone who is thoughtful, quiet and controlled). If, however, you are an extravert (active, sociable and impulsive) you are likely to forget the unfortunate lover, toiling away, lovelorn, back at home and instead make a rapid recovery, filling up your life with interesting new acquaintances.

And that's more likely to happen if you are attractive. The more attractive your appearance, the more people will fall for you, offer you good jobs and want to be your friend. The research bears this out. Take a look at the colleagues in your office and keep in mind that all around you have been chosen because they appeal (in some way) to the male or female executive doing the hiring.

THE MYTHS OF ROMANTIC LOVE

There are many beliefs about romantic love that psychological research has shown to be unfounded. Here are four of the most common ones.

myth: Women fall in love more easily than men do.
truth: Women tend to fall in love with men after the men have fallen in love first.

myth: Men are much more likely to leave a marriage than women are.
truth: Divorce statistics show that far more women than men end marriages

myth: Men don't like women to make the first moves in a relationship.
truth: Men welcome enthusiastic attention.

myth: Fascinating, exotic strangers end up with the most desirable mates.
truth: We are most likely to get it together with the boy or the girl next door. We prefer someone who is familiar and with whom we have been able to enjoy casual easy contact at first.

THE ROMEO AND JULIET SYNDROME

Yes, but suppose you fall in love with someone who, once the romance has worn off, is unsuitable? What can you do? Firstly a warning to parents. The Romeo and Juliet syndrome appears to show that the worst thing you can do is object to your offspring's unsuitable partner. Objection produces hothouse conditions for love and actually fertilises passion. The only way for one partner to discover the true unworthiness of the other is by living through the initial romance, painful though it may be. The consolation is that, since we generally learn from experience, we won't make the same mistake again.

THE BIOLOGY OF LOVE

We tend to assume that everybody regards love in the same all-consuming fashion, as a pointer to existence, as a signpost for the way in which we live life. This isn't, however, the case. Psychologists refer to love as infatuation and declare that other societies, recognising its temporary status, organise their social lives *despite* it, rather than as a *result* of it. Biology, however, needs men and women to get together sexually for the continuation of the species. Love, thus a part of evolutionary design, works by rewarding the individual with a love cocktail, an adrenaline rush made up of hormones (dopamine, noradrenaline and a large component of phenylethylamine (PEA)).

This chemical concoction creates an altered state of consciousness. People will say and do things in this mind-state, that they wouldn't in normal circumstances. Mental defences are lowered. People get a glimpse of a different side to themselves. They say things like 'I've never been able to talk like this to anyone before'. Similarities between lovers are highlighted and differences appear negligible. They want to spend all their time together and friends become suddenly less important.

Please note:
- Love allows us to become more open to the other.
- Love lets us trust because we see only good.
- Love lets you believe that you want the same things.

The reason why we reiterate these points is that good *sex* may also let you think these things. In fact, there's a strong chance that love and

THE LOVE PLAN

1 **Open up to each other.**
Deliberately opening up to a partner, as we've discussed in the previous chapter, fosters trust and gives a platform on which to form the relationship.

2 **Match stories and experiences.**
Deliberately matching personal stories fosters liking and a sense of security.

3 **Think obsessively about the other.**
Thinking non-stop about the other person heightens intensity, arousal and the sexual outcome.

sex are circular, each leading to the other in certain favourable circumstances. Many people do *not* love a partner to begin with but find that the sex is good and so begin to fall in love. Out of this inter-twining of love and sex therefore we note some particular factors that foster love. If we understand how falling in love actually works, we gain some extra options such as the ability to place ourselves in love's path or out of it.

So far, so good. All of this is wonderful and exciting. But falling in love also involves a blending of personality and a blending of emotions. Suddenly you feel you *are* the other person. Yet if you 'are' that person, how can you know what is them and what is you? Suppose you have a penchant for bondage and submission? How can you be sure that your loved one thinks similarly? How can you know that you aren't just projecting your own enthusiasms onto her unreciprocating libido?

The problem with falling madly in love is that choice becomes blended. Your choice feels like theirs. What's more, they want it to be so. Just how do you disentangle which one of you is which? And while you are doing this, how do you avoid making a poor sexual judgement that will ultimately erect barriers between you? Women, like men, need to feel they can make their own choices. What you never want to do is pressure a partner into acting out things that she radically dislikes

LEARNING LOVE SKILLS

The **first** comfort is to remember that it is human to make mistakes – we all do it. And nowhere are we more likely to do so than in the delicate

Mike, a 37 year old doctor, described the first weeks of a new relationship that evolved into a long term one. 'In retrospect, all the things that I found very difficult later on were there in the beginning. We were madly in love, having a wonderful sex life, but she just didn't turn up for dates. By the time I'd gone through stages of disappointment, anger and then withdrawal, she would finally arrive, sometimes three hours later, looking perfectly comfortable, saying 'Well, I met Bob by accident and I knew you wouldn't mind if I spent some time with him, because you see me all the time and he hardly sees me at all'. She didn't think she'd done anything wrong.

'I managed to get her to improve in that she would actually give me some warning when she wasn't going to be on time and meanwhile I was so blinded by love that I honestly thought I could manage. But it emerged that she was also sleeping with these friends. And after a two and half year relationship I woke up one day and thought 'this is ridiculous. I'm in pain a lot of the time. She isn't going to change.' To this day, she thinks I'm mad for giving up on what she considered a wonderful committed loving relationship. What started off small, became a very big obstacle for me in the end.'

balance of love and sex. The **second** is to find out as much as you can about her background. This is on the grounds that, by picking up a sense of the pattern that she and her family operates by emotionally, you will get some idea of how to weave her differences in with yours. The **third is** that bearing in mind it's hard to recognise such differences, tell yourself firmly that even small things matter and take precautions, even if they seem virtually unnecessary at the time.

The **fourth** rule of thumb is to always take things slowly at the beginning of establishing good sex. If she's nervous and inhibited she'll thank you for it. If she's impatient and in a rush, she'll be tantalised, and if she's highly sexed she'll either make the running herself or respond with massively increased sensuality.

AFTER THE CHEMICAL RUSH IS OVER

One of the places where biology got it wrong is that the addictive chemical rush that assaults your senses so pleasingly in the first months begins to wear off. It is annoyingly time-dependent and, depending on how often you've fallen in love before, dwindles after the third or the sixth month. If you had previously thought the other person was magic, you may suddenly see them as having gone seriously off. You question their true colours, which is hard on them, when you should also be questioning *yours*.

GETTING ATTACHED

Why should you question yourself? Think of a love relationship as possessing three specific phases. The first is **attraction**, the second is **infatuation** and the third, which happens when the honeymoon phase ends, is **attachment**. People who enjoyed secure attachment to their parents when they were children, won't find it difficult to move on from infatuation to attachment. They will instinctively know how to do attachment behaviour because they will have unconsciously taken in the model they experienced at home.

Such behaviours encourage the giving and receiving of love, they allow the sensuality of sex gratification, the self-calming and soothing that is sometimes necessary in moments of upset. That is because these behaviours provoke a different set of chemicals, in this case an endorphin response, which produces calm, peace, a sense of security.

If your woman friend has not displayed the above characteristics, it may be you, in your eagerness, who has misjudged, rather than she who has misled. Perhaps you have read soothing and supportive characteristics into her because you wanted to see them there. However before you give up on her totally, why not try to understand why she might not display attachment behaviours?

Let's suppose that your woman friend has *not* had the experience of secure parental attachment. Suppose at heart she feels unlovable because that's what childhood has left her with? This means that she may be able to give love but not be too brilliant at receiving it. It means that because she doesn't really believe in your love *she begins to test you*. Each test grows increasingly hard and somewhere along the line you're bound to fail, if only to a small degree, not surprisingly since you won't have the faintest idea why she is doing this. (Neither, incidentally, will she.)

THE PAIN OF SEPARATION

Believing that you are failing her, she goes into *a defence mode of mentally separating* from you. John Bowlby, developer of the attachment theory, based his notions on studies of children who were separated from their parents. He observed that they went through three phases:

1 The children **protested.**
2 Next, they grieved and grew **despondent.**
3 Finally, they looked as if they were getting over the loss. They played with other children or with toys. What actually happened was they **separated** themselves from their pain, by building a wall of protection.

Grown-ups do the same. If you start to get frantic, or blaming, or really bad-tempered you're probably in the **protest** stage. If your partner does nothing to reassure, you begin to feel quite despairing about the long-term survival for the relationship. And if still no real contact or reassurance takes place, you galvanise yourself into action. You rally your friends round for support, you take yourself out and socialise with others, you immerse yourself in a new absorbing project – in other words you distance yourself.

The good news is that even at this stage the relationship can improve. All it takes is a kind overture from a partner and you feel

ATTACHMENT BEHAVIOURS

These include:

❦ supporting

❦ holding

❦ touching

❦ gazing

❦ co-operating

❦ negotiating

❦ listening

❦ responding

❦ validating

❦ comforting

better. A bit more conversation and you start feeling secure again. A bit more soothing, in the shape of physical comfort and you get back on line – you regain attachment.

Most of us experience the aforementioned scenario, if only mildly. So what should you do about it? At least one of you needs a recognition method so that you can intercept and interpret her distress signals. You also need the belief that the distress doesn't necessarily mean the end of the relationship but rather that you need to *renew the connection*.

DISTRESS SIGNALS CODE

1 **Signal:** Partner gets cranky, argumentative, and picks on you.
Code: She is worried stiff about something emotional that she considers to be not working with you. The complication is that this may have absolutely nothing to do with you but derive largely from her own childhood.
Cue: Find out her core feeling and where it comes from. Give her reassurance.

2 **Signal:** Partner goes all quiet, withdraws from arguments, or walks away from them refusing to be drawn in any longer. You catch her weeping and looking quite hopeless.
Code: She's giving up and retreating into depression.
Cue: Stop arguing and listen to her feelings. Instead of getting self-defensive recognise that certain childhood buttons of hers, which have nothing to do with you, have been pushed. See if you can identify what they are and pay attention to them. It's no good dismissing them on the grounds that they aren't relevant in the here and now – unfortunately they continue to function. Acknowledge verbally that these are distressing her and ask her to work on ways on which to alter her mindset. Offer to go some of the way to changing your behaviour (even if this seems unreasonable). Unless you are prepared to make some change, she won't feel that you are sincere. And give her physical and verbal reassurance.

3 **Signal:** Partner is suddenly never at home in the evening, appears to have become a workaholic and is so absorbed by a new-found interest in fund-raising for the Hospital Trust, that you just never see her.

Code: She is distancing herself from the pain she feels in your presence by finding other interests that take her mind off her unhappiness at home.

Cue: Make a date with her to talk since it no longer happens spontaneously even in the shape of fights. If necessary, make a date with a counsellor. And then follow the cue for Signal 2. Supplement the discussion with massive verbal and physical reassurance.

It's no accident that we have emphasised the role of reassurance. What you are dealing with here is someone who feels discouraged and hopeless, even though you can't for the life of you see why. Until you can recognise and acknowledge it, you can't help her. But change is needed. And you, uncomfortable though it seems, will also have to change. You will need to interpret her behaviour regularly and accurately and grasp her real goal, which is to be loved, because of and in spite of herself. You will need to read between the lines of bad behaviour and offer her reassurance rather than flak.

SEX AND ENCOURAGEMENT

Where does sex fit into attachment? One theory has it that relationships contain only a few emotional milestones. These include falling in love, experiencing the birth of our children and dealing with death. (Of course, if we are unlucky there may be other terrible milestones but these are more likely to detach us than foster closeness.) Sex therefore may be the cement that bonds us together between emotional events, the glue that keeps the relationship happy. It also gives some very inhibited human beings permission to touch. And touch, as previously discussed, is vital to calming us, to offering a sense of value and of love – keeping the peace.

However, sex is hard to enjoy if you're feeling bad. Although anger can provide a temporary high and result in explosive sex, too much anger can seriously erode affection and trust grows ever more difficult to seek.

Touch demonstrates physically the words 'I love you', soothes upset, restores self-value and is integral to true sensuality. True sensuality *cannot exist* without knowledge of touch. Some people appear to be touch masters by instinct, responding to a partner's needs apparently by osmosis. For others, touching skills need to be learned.

Don't panic. We have ways of making you appear a touch master even at the first attempt.

TWENTY WAYS TO TOUCH A LOVER

1 Make sure your hands are warm and dry.

2 Make sure the room is warm.

3 Touch slowly and deliberately.

4 Never touch suddenly – never plonk a hand heavily on your lover's body.

5 Offer distinct strokes such as in a massage.

6 Only stroke fleshy areas.

7 Never stroke on bone.

8 Stroke away from the spine – never towards it.

9 Don't let strokes be only sensual ones, let touch convey friendship too. That is, use touch in friendly situations.

10 Vary the pressure of your strokes. Understand that different pressures offer different impressions.

11 A firm stroke offers matter-of-factness and a sense of security.

12 A lighter stroke indicates playfulness and hints at sensuality.

13 A fingertips-only stroke is meltingly arousing.

14 A fingernails-only stroke is outright X-rated.

ONLY A HAND

A good beginning is to place a hand on your lover's body. It's a simple move. But it's *how* you place the hand, where you place it, the warmth and firmness of your touch that all contribute a tactile impression.

15 If, when you get to bed, a massage seems a good preliminary, all of the above apply, plus the expediency of using warm massage oil.

16 Different massages have differing degrees of security/insecurity. The routine offering the safest feeling is a foot massage.

17 Another non-threatening routine is a head massage. You might do this while shampooing, where you massage your lover's scalp through the suds.

18 A hair massage. This can be a part of a head massage or totally separate. It tends to feel best when fingertips have stimulated the scalp first. Take a small tuft of hair between your fingertips and tug on it gently a couple of times. Repeat this movement with tufts from all over, until you have completely covered the head.

19 Any massage, be it head or full body, benefits from a variation of the circling stroke. You can do this with the whole hand or with the fingertips. You can make large slow circles on the back or buttocks and small slow circles on the scalp.

CASE HISTORY

Paul was first attracted to Jenny in a meeting at her home, before her imminent divorce. While the group chatted, Jenny caressed her little daughter. Paul was unable to take his eyes off her hands. 'I could see from the way she touched that little girl that this was a very sensual lady,' he told us. Acting on his observation Paul asked Jenny round for a massage. She turned up not really believing he was serious. He was. He oiled and creamed and smoothed her skin for nearly an hour, paying attention to every hungry inch. When she finally and with difficulty sat upright again, she felt liking and affection for him that was completely unlike ordinary sexual desire, perhaps because she was utterly relaxed in spite of sitting there naked.

After a short time she decided she would like to return the favour. This time, she massaged Paul. He was extremely sexually aroused by the experience but made no attempt to initiate intercourse, being willing to accept the massage for the sake of good touch alone. Jenny felt so empowered by the obvious success of her ministrations and by the knowledge that she appeared to be in charge of this experience that she couldn't resist initiating sex. She was usually very tense when making love for the first time and unable to climax. This occasion was different. 'She took ages to come but it didn't matter – it felt like part of the massage,' Paul told us. 'Good sensations just built up and up – I was playing a game with myself to *stop* me from coming. It felt as if we'd known each other for years.' In Jenny and Paul's case the massage was the beginning of a passionate long-term love-affair.

TOUCH AND THE MECHANICS OF ATTRACTION

A university team, researching the ingredients of love and attraction found that visual and tactile warmth moves rated highly.

Included in the list were:

- He looks into her eyes
- Touches her hand
- Moves towards her
- Smiles frequently
- Works his eyes from her head to her toes
- Has a happy smile, grins,
- Uses expressive hand gestures when speaking

20 To get an idea of how touch is feeling to your partner close your eyes, as your hands contact her skin, and experience your own sensations. How does it feel to you? Does a different pressure, or slowing down make the action more sensual for you? If it does, the odds are it will for her too.

Anne's somewhat eccentric opinion has it that if we were all encouraged to give and receive a massage daily, aggression, vandalism, delinquency and war would rapidly diminish.

TOUCH GAMES

Ray Stubbs in the 1970s was a legendary master of massage in San Francisco. Here are three touch games that Ray used to recommend to his pupils.

The first is the **Touch Me Test**, where couples stroke tiny sections of each other's bodies and rate their reactions on a score of plus or minus three. It sounds crazy and ends up feeling wonderful. The most unexpected areas, such as under the big toe, can rate plus 10! And after the laughter and embarrassment have died down, it is highly effective for allowing couples to learn (sometimes for the first time) which areas of their partner are most sexually responsive.

The second game is **Rag Doll**, where one partner remains completely limp while the other manipulates her limbs in any way he thinks is desirable.

The third is the **Pampered Foot**. Here the recipients find to their amazement that their most sensual area isn't between the legs but way down at the end of them. The Pampered Foot is a cross between a foot-bath and a foot massage. You need a bowl of warm water, a bottle of liquid soap and a pair of warm, supple and flexible hands.

EVERYDAY SENSUALITY

If games aren't your scene, try building up the sensuality that already exists between you by always:

- Cuddling in the morning when you wake up
- Kissing as you pass each other in the kitchen
- Patting on the bottom when you do the washing up
- Putting an arm around her shoulders or her waist when you work on something together
- Holding a hand (or even a foot) as you watch television together
- Putting your arms around her from the back and leaning her in towards your body when you make conversation with a third party
- Augmenting touch with the phrase 'I love you'.

SEX AND INTIMACY

Sex is a core ingredient of intimacy, although not the only one. The very act of sex, even if it's with a stranger, means that we leave ourselves intensely vulnerable for a short time. Good sex opens us up in a flower-like sense letting us appreciate the qualities of the person who has drawn such wonderful feelings to the surface. Although good sex and love are not necessarily inter-related, very often they are. One promotes the other. Sex provides a short cut to a lover's personality. If sex goes wrong, this may be a signpost to other aspects of the relationship. Some people, women in particular, feel you can only have good sex with people you love.

So we return to the beginning – love matters to most women. By placing yourself in its path, by developing uncanny skills of diagnosing emotional compatibility and by tuning in to her skin with your finger-tips, you've given yourself a head start.

THE ARTS OF good sex

Here's where things get really physical. This is the part of the book that teaches you to stir up sensation under every inch of her skin. You've wooed her and won. She's crazy about you. She's dying to make mad passionate love with you. Go for it.

FEMALE PYROTECHNICS

Think of the feminine form as a swirl of erotic energy. Picture clouds of electric particles sizzling through the pores of her skin and firing up towards the sky. This is your woman's erotic potential. This is her ability to light up with such power that every inch of her form wants to glow and sing. OK, we're talking figuratively. Yet, some people believe that the skin actually possesses an electrical potential that can illuminate a torch battery!

DEEP DOWN INSIDE

Women who report being able to react as Shirley did say that this is *not* something that happens with any regularity. It's an occasional special high. One of the defining features is a particular throbbing sensation experienced deep down. The sensation described corresponds to sex researchers Masters and Johnson's mention of 'pelvic throbbing' in the womb (more of this later). This throbbing is equated with high levels of excitement and may be particularly noticeable when the entire body has reached an ecstatic sensual pitch. On the grounds that it is analogous to extreme arousal, we researched the subject to help *your* woman towards it.

PELVIC THROBBING – THE RESEARCH

1 The Orgasmic Platform: In their observations of female orgasm, sex researchers Masters and Johnson described a concept that they call the 'orgasmic platform'. This is part of the initial build up of sensual tension in the vagina – a normal stage in the excitement process. The first sign of excitement amounts to a type of vaginal dilation or widening. As the dilation continues, the back section of the vagina opens. The inside of the vagina, at the far end, expands till it 'tents' – turning itself into a mini-cavern – and this is the 'orgasmic platform'.

2 Tenting: The condition of 'tenting', or holding the orgasmic platform, can continue for a long time. It is no guarantee of orgasm although it is most definitely the launch pad. It takes just a little more stimulation before the take-off into climax can begin.

3 Throbbing: Many women report that, *before* the climax actually moves into repeated vaginal contractions, they experience pelvic *throbbing*. The throbbing is *not* experienced as a vaginal contraction although the two may soon become merged. We think that throbbing is probably a rhythm of extreme excitement – mini or internal contractions. Meanwhile, more easily recognised external orgasmic contractions take place in the outer two-thirds of the vagina (which is not 'tented' but very swollen with desire).

So, just to make it absolutely clear, *women can experience two different types of orgasmic contraction, both sequentially and simultaneously.*

Masters and Johnson equated pelvic throbbing with 'recurring orgasmic-platform contractions'. In other words, they actually managed to observe the throbbing in the 'tented' area. What's more, they say that the consciousness of pulsations frequently continues beyond the observable 'platform' contractions. Perhaps – and this is pure surmise – perhaps the completely excited and aroused female is capable of being aroused in every part of her sexual anatomy – even that which is situated deep inside her, such as her uterus. Masters and Johnson's work with pregnant women shows clearly that the pregnant uterus contracts noticeably during sex, sometimes with much greater strength than it did before pregnancy.

Our hypothesis is that it may be possible to create such pelvic throbbing by using concentrated body friction plus kissing prior to intercourse; and that since clitoral or vaginal stimulation is not yet taking place, the throbbing may happen over and over again.

If a certain type of arousal is needed to create the platform and make it 'throb' what might that be? We'll make some educated guesses shortly. Do all women experience this vaginal throbbing? We don't know. Might all women possess the potential for vaginal throbbing? We don't know that either but readers of this book can have fun finding out.

What the well-informed lover needs to know is that he may be able to stir his woman to the very depths of her body and soul by 1) the art of kissing 2) stimulating her brain and 3) close all-over body contact.

1. THE ART OF KISSING

We seem to have forgotten about the power of kissing in the West in the 21st century. The ancient *Kama Sutra*, written at the beginning of the Christian calendar, devoted dozens of paragraphs to the subject. Kissing was taken very seriously indeed by the illustrious author, and soft kisses, passionate kisses, tongue-to-tongue experiences all possessed specific

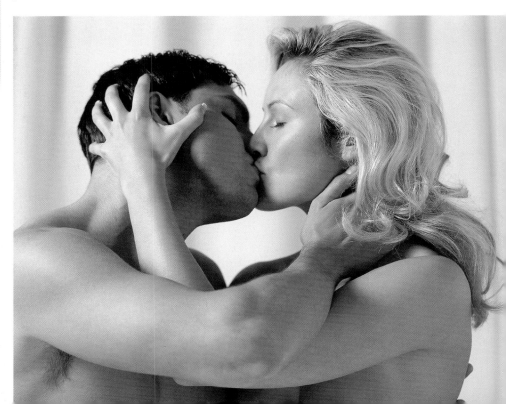

meaning. We feel that it is right to treat kissing in such detail because it is capable of so many things. It can demonstrate how a love affair is likely to progress. It can stimulate passion and be a marker of great love. Done with skill and variety it can be a sensual, exciting experience in its own right. If you thought kissing was an unimportant preliminary, merely a component of foreplay, you've missed out on a wealth of erotic sensation. If you thought that there's little to it, you're in for a pleasant surprise. Even if you're one who doesn't like kissing, let's give you a chance to re-think your resistance.

HOW TO KISS

Yael's list offers some clues. There's the:

1 Very shy, very young kiss where the lips are merely pressed together without much movement. If your woman shows little response or little movement of her own lips, take things very slowly indeed. She's only learning.

2 Testing-out kiss consisting of a very light explorative touch, touching only briefly, then withdrawing, but then re-alighting once more as if to say 'that felt so good that I'd like to experience more'. This can be repeated many times but only if she responds by moving her own lips.

3 Light kiss on the side of the mouth, repeated in a little shower of touch all around her lips. These are kisses that show affection and liking.

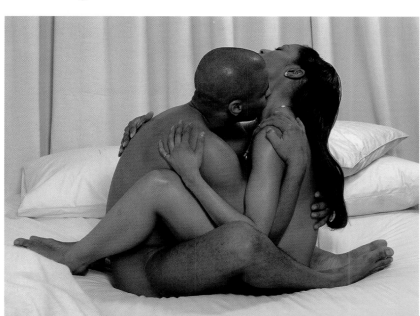

YAEL'S STORY

'When my present lover kissed me for the first time I started off by thinking 'Oh, what a drag.' But the kiss turned out to be magic. To start with it was very light and soft – it didn't feel intrusive or invasive. I knew I wouldn't have to endure anything I didn't want to. But more happened. Because his lips were so light on mine, I could experience every small movement of them and it was as if he were transmitting some wonderfully held-back but intense moment of passion. I couldn't help responding. I kissed back instead of just letting it happen. And he kissed me in turn. And then I kissed once more. And the pressure of our lips, which had started off like the touching of clouds, got firmer as we fell into a new dimension. I also felt little electric shocks, like static off a light switch.

'Every time we stopped one of us felt compelled to go back for more and the kisses got harder and more urgent. They also got more explorative. I remember biting him slightly and finding that his mouth opened in a kind of helplessness. It was as if we ran through an entire love affair in the space of 10 minutes kissing. It took me from being totally uninterested to longing for him.'

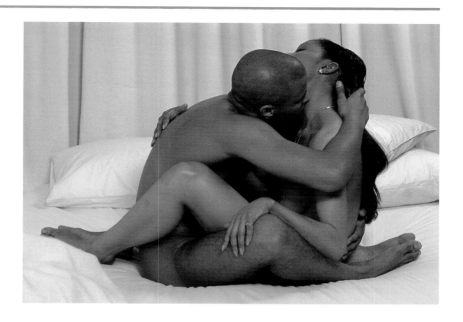

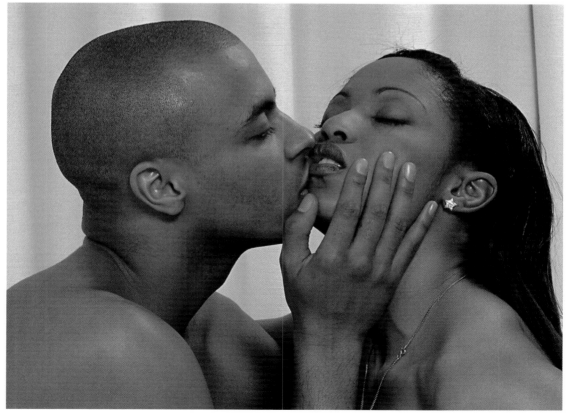

4 Slightly firmer kiss, (but not hard) that indicates you find her very attractive.

5 Long-lasting kiss where you let the insides of your mouth melt into the insides of hers. She will need to open her mouth slightly to let this happen. You might try gently nudging it open with the movement of your mouth. But never force things. Always let kissing flow.

6 Very slight tongue probe, simply on and around her lips. Using your tongue indicates a further degree of intimacy and needs to be done slowly, gradually. If you ever feel her recoil take the hint. This means you have gone too far, too fast. Withdraw a little to something less pressured.

7 The passionate kiss. As you sense her getting more aroused don't be afraid of making the kisses even firmer. The firmer the kiss the more aroused is the signal.

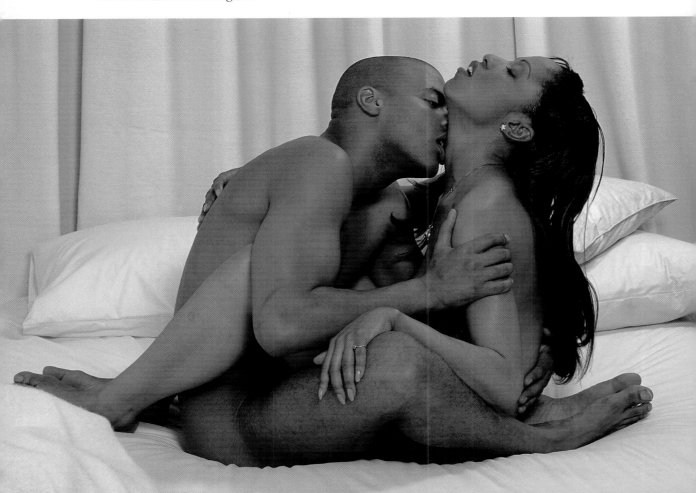

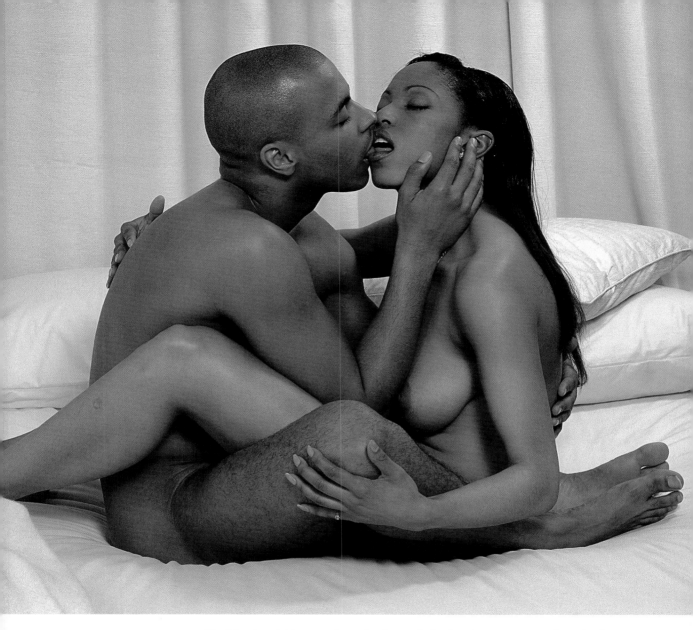

8 The hard kiss – only to be hazarded when you are sure that she is
   aroused. Usually to be done at the end of a sequence of kissing.
   But on exceptional occasions to be done immediately, provided
   you know you are completely hot for each other.

9 Biting. This is a very excited version of hard kissing and indicates
   that you are so aroused by her that you want to possess her
   utterly. Don't do it with any serious intent to wound. Just take
   little nips, hard enough to sting but not hard enough to hurt.

It should have become clear from the above that kissing starts off soft and continues through firm to hard, and in so doing, echoes what goes on genitally. Indeed, it sometimes seems that there is a direct connection between mouth and vagina since passionate kissing can cause pelvic spasms and internal 'throbbing'. It can literally make your knees feel weak and your legs turn to jelly. And yes, kissing alone can cause that pelvic throbbing. The more subtly and variously you manage it, the more aroused she should become.

HOW NOT TO KISS

There are however, some very specific ways in which you should *not* kiss. You should not:

- *Force* your tongue down her throat – ever.
- Push her or hurt her with your mouth.
- Start with hard kissing since this can be interpreted as a hostile act.
- Push the progress of kissing. If she recoils or rejects, accept that you have gone too far and withdraw.

Kissing should not be invasive, but exploratory. It should not be aggressive, but eager. Kissing is not about inflicting your attentions on someone, but about provoking a delightful response. If you ever doubt what effect your kissing is having, close your eyes and concentrate on the experience your own lips receive. If you sense that there is very little feeling you are probably going at things too hard and anaesthetising your own pleasure.

Kissing doesn't work with everyone. People don't always respond in the way you recognise, don't pick up the signals you try to give. Often it boils down to chemistry. If the chemistry isn't right, kissing can be a direct way of registering this. Many people believe that you can diagnose a person's intimate nature from the way he or she kisses. It's a useful exercise to ask yourself, next time you pucker your lips towards an attractive face, just what you might be telling her about yourself.

Kissing is the very first part of sex and an integral part. Skimp on the kissing and you send an instant message that good sex is probably not going to be very high on your agenda.

A very few women report being able to climax through fantasy alone. Janet revealed: 'I used to lie in bed next to my husband whom I didn't love and with whom I had rarely climaxed. I would remain completely still so that I didn't disturb him and think of my lover. I would remember the sexy stories he used to tell me in bed, would get hugely aroused and would end up having orgasms in complete silence, without deliberately moving a muscle. I did this once standing at a bus stop, and actually climaxed in the street, without another soul knowing.'

2. STIMULATING HER BRAIN

There can be a right way and a wrong way to do this. At its height, sexy talk can turn some women on just by ideas but you can also convey similar ideas with physical moves.

SEX TALK

Some people feel uncomfortable using sexual language. If this is a major part of your partner's turn-on, how can you compensate?

There is a Californian sex therapy exercise in which clients are:

- Encouraged to collect all the sexual words they can think of.
- Requested to stand in front of a full-length mirror and read the words out loud.
- Asked, with each reading, to increase the volume, until they are shouting.
- Asked to repeat the exercise in front of a partner. With reassurance and encouragement from the partner, it works.

That's one way forward.

You can also convey sensual ideas by telling sexual stories and describing fantasy scenarios. (See Chapter Eight on storytelling.)

THE MIND IS SOVEREIGN

We don't know exactly what happens when women like Janet stimulate themselves purely through the power of thought but we can take an educated guess. Erotic thoughts probably persuade the brain to send messages of arousal to the genitals. The messages are powerful enough and persistent enough to build up excitement culminating in the 'plateau phase', or 'orgasmic platform'. Where Janet is different from

SEX FACTS FROM MASTERS & JOHNSON'S RESEARCH

- Lesbians giving their partners oral stimulation climaxed themselves without receiving direct genital stimulation.

- Physiological evidence showed that, with all subjects, the longer and more teasing the build-up, the more aroused the person being stimulated the deeper the subsequent experience of orgasm.

many other women is that she possesses enough mental power of self-excitement to nudge herself up off the orgasmic platform, right into the throes of orgasm.

Other women report similar experiences but describe the culmination as 'not actually orgasm, but such intense excitement that I'm on the edge, throbbing and pulsating genitally.' The real point is that the mind is a totally powerful stimulant where women are concerned, responding immediately to suggestion as well as to all-over body contact.

It almost goes without saying that, if there are loving and effective ways to turn women on, there are also unpleasant sexual events that can ultimately turn women off. Research work carried out in West Germany showed that, although both sexes grew aroused by films depicting rape, women showed *stronger turn-off reactions* than men. It may be possible to read from this that gentler approaches to sex have a better effect on women even though they are capable of being aroused by emotionally extreme sexual visuals.

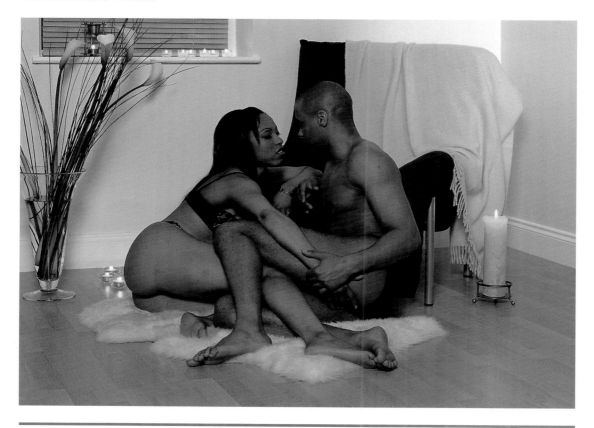

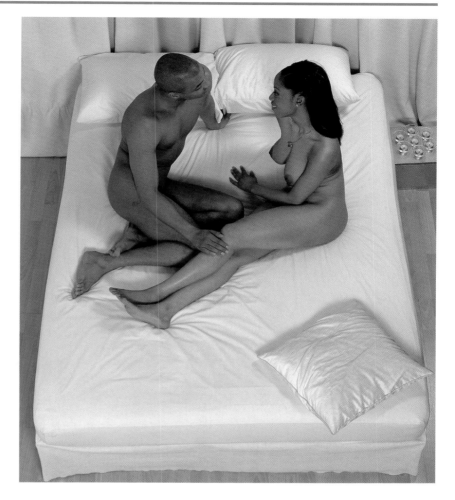

Fantasy collections show marked sex difference in content. Men tend to prefer harder core fantasies, which are specifically sexual. Many women, by contrast, find scenes of floating in lapping oceans and melting into golden sunsets arousing.

Of course, there are always exceptions: we know women who like pain, ritual sado-masochism and domination for their sexual diet. But we also know many more women who adore the romantic approach, would give anything to be glamorously wooed and who respond to the slow but sensual approach above all others. It's the latter we are focusing on here. Making physical moves that convey tender warmth are the most certain way of nurturing her belief that you are a sexy, erotic individual who is magically tuning in to her very feminine wavelength.

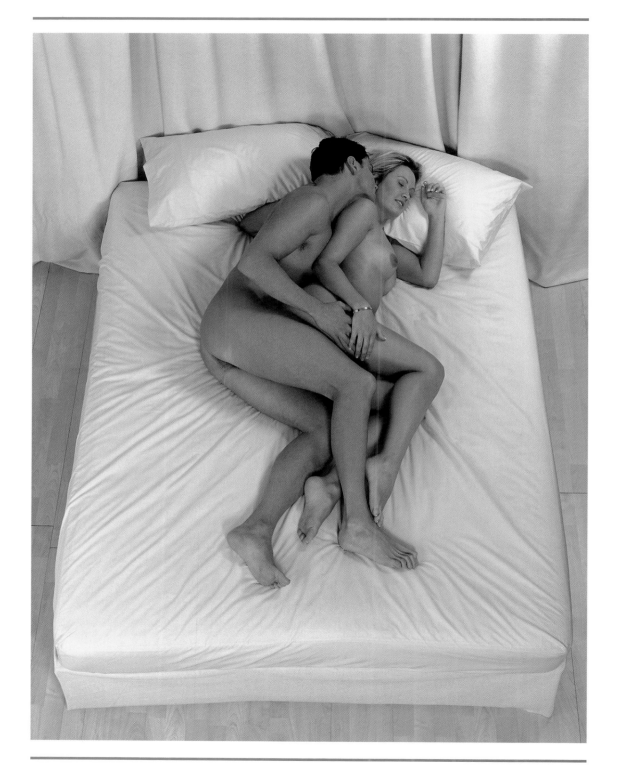

EROTIC IDEAS

Once wonderful kissing has established your credentials as an erotic personality it's time to heighten the passion further. As you stagger towards the bed, drunk with desire, you suddenly remember that Woody Allen's ambition was to possess Warren Beatty's fingertips. Here are some suggestions for the kind of master patterns that Mr Beatty's fingers might have traced on bodies too numerous to list:

- Kiss and gently bite her neck.
- Work your way up the neck towards her ear.
- Nibble and nuzzle her ear (but avoid making it wet).
- Breathe deliberately (but quietly) into her ear.
- Stroke her lips with your fingers as you kiss her.
- Take her hand in yours and idly circle the palm with your fingertips.
- As you kiss her, cradling her head with one hand, let your free hand stroke and caress her body.
- Tell her you find her incredibly attractive.
- Turn her back towards you and kiss into the nape of her neck.
- Prolong the kissing there and turn it into soft biting.

TAKING OFF HER CLOTHES

Trying to kiss her while struggling with the fastenings of her clothes is not sexy. Either make up your mind to make love with all your clothes on or deliberately focus on undressing her without the distraction of carrying on the caresses.

- You might suggest that she talks you through unbuttoning and disrobing her.
- You could try removing her clothes in stages, spending a good 15 minutes on each portion of her anatomy revealed.
- Best of all is to kiss her into such a daze that she unconsciously starts shedding garments that just happen to get in the way!

In general, being deliberate about undressing rather than trying to do it unobtrusively and failing miserably is the best way to handle a new lover. It may sound odd to be so dictatorial about how to undress your woman but the process is rooted in the notion of psychological impact.

Every move you make, the way in which you handle potentially sensitive situations such as taking off clothes, creates an impression. And that impression affects whether or not she gets hotter and hotter.

NUDITY INHIBITIONS

Many women are nervous about showing their naked body because they believe that they are ugly. These beliefs may be left over from a verbally abusive parent or boyfriend. Sometimes such feelings are part of depression. One woman, Katie, taking part in Anne's sexuality groups, had the utmost difficulty stripping in order to participate in the massage session. She looked awful, she said, and was covered in acne. She endured the massage by retaining items of underwear, yet by the time the massage had ended she felt so differently that she was able to cast these off too. We could see that her skin was virtually flawless. This woman went on to make major changes in her life, having been paralysed by depression for two years.

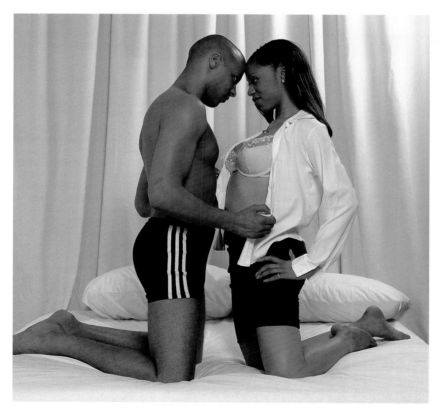

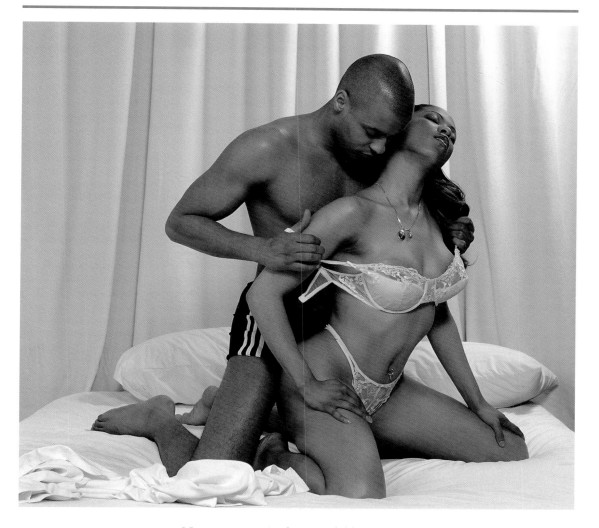

Not everyone is depressed like Katie but many will recognise the anxiety about displaying a body that they consider to be less than perfect. So, move with care and consideration. Women are self-conscious about their bodies and sometimes find it difficult to cope with being watched. Try to arrange the lighting so that it is soft and discreet – candles are definitely the sexiest option. Incidentally, when *you* are undressing and wish to ensure that she sees you at your most attractive make damn sure you take your socks off *first*. She may not be aware of it but everything about her surroundings will impinge on her feelings of sensuality. How you look, how you undress, how the room smells, how warm or cold it is, all of this will encourage or discourage her response.

3. CLOSE BODY CONTACT

And when you've got her there, on the bed, in all her naked glory, what next?

MORE EROTIC IDEAS

Snuggle together as if you are kids. You don't have to start off by kissing. If undressing has proved something of an interruption, don't feel

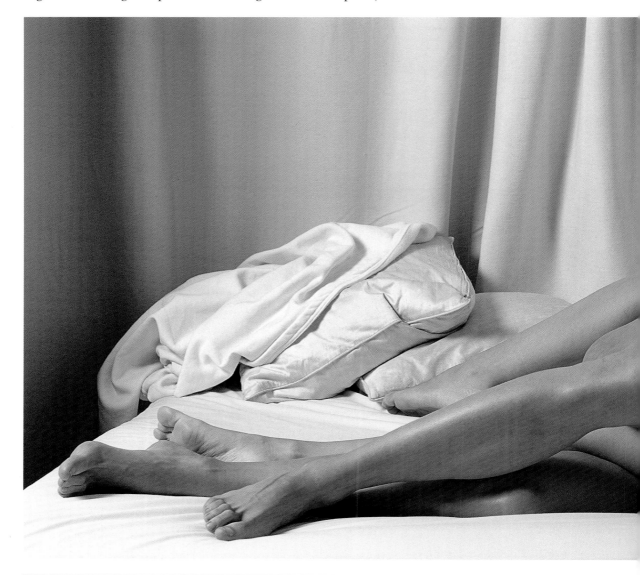

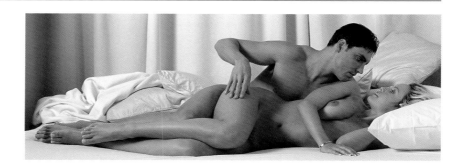

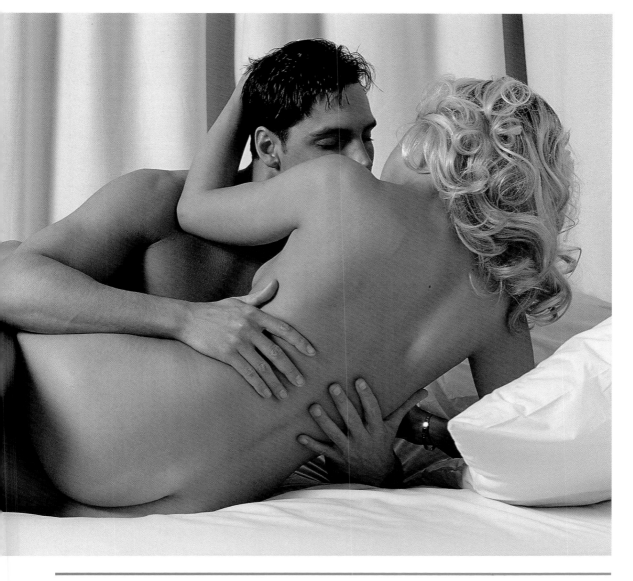

you have to take up exactly where you left off. It's probably better to consider that you have entered a new phase where lying down is the new beginning.

- Cuddling
- Snuggling
- Lying in the spoons position
- Playing
- Finger-tipping across each other's body
- Back-scratching with lightly placed well-smoothed fingernails
- Stroking the breasts, the belly, the tops of the legs
- Accidentally brushing against her labia with your fingers
- The more you stroke, the more you accidentally brush
- Stroke her lips, as you kiss, with one hand and with the other, begin to stroke her clitoris – a two-pronged attack
- Try combinations of stroking the top half of the body with one hand and the genitals with the other.

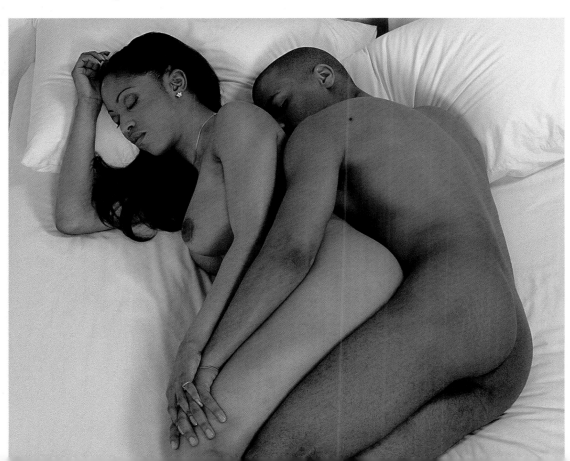

LET LIGHTNING STRIKE

Flicking, licking, breathing, sliding, these have to be the ingredients of oral sex. Forty years ago nice middle-class girls didn't know it existed but then came a book called *The Sensuous Woman* by 'J'. And the revelation that made the name of this innovative if anonymous volume was the chapter on How to do Fellatio. Suddenly, women were exploring techniques to practise on their men such as the 'butterfly flick' and the 'ice cream swirl' while delighted lovers were teased to the point of explosion. What follows here is role reversal. We list a number of tantalising oral sex techniques for men to bedazzle their women.

CUNNING LINGUISM

There are few sexual activities so personal, so intimate, so totally accepting. If you want your woman to feel validated as the most sensuous

PERSONAL STORY

Frances explained to us that her partner often moves on to oral sex after the two of them have cuddled and stroked and massaged first so that their bodies are already sexually energised.

'He eases my legs open and slides his shoulders under them. Then he presses my vaginal lips together and kisses them with the whole of his mouth. I feel warm, damp and excited. He opens me up with his tongue and probes gently along the inside of my outer vaginal lips, moving from the clitoris towards the far end.

'The inner lips are sucked gently into his mouth and licked one at a time. His tongue slides over the whole length of me and then curves gently inside for a few damp, velvet moments. I think, please let him touch my clit now. And he does. His fingers open me right up, pushing back the outer lips and, with the very tip of his tongue, he eases back the hood and presses down so that it stands out. He sucks me right into his mouth as his lips close around it.

'His tongue flicks at and circles the top of my clitoris, more and more quickly. And the sucking continues. I can feel my own heat, the swelling of my entire vaginal area and I hear, from far off, my own soft moans.

'Slowly he pushes his finger into my vagina: I can feel my own smooth wetness. His fingers move in and out slowly as his tongue vibrates relentlessly against my clit. He's taking me there. I feel hardly conscious, lost in unbearable tension as my pleasure builds up and tightens into a rhythmic series of contractions that go on and on.'

representative of her sex, cunnilingus is the means. This is not some knockabout foreplay – you are employing a precision process as flexible and as versatile as tongue (and fingers) can be. It provides a moistness, a dexterity, a pointed exactitude that bigger clumsier caresses can never achieve. It is an instrument that might have been designed for the tiny bud that is your lover's sexual pleasure centre. Hear Frances' description of her lover's tantalising technique.

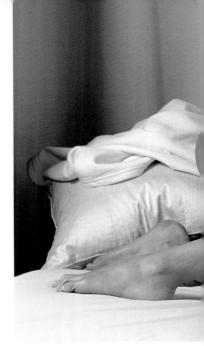

GETTING INTO TRAINING

Tongue twisters. Exercise your 'organ of exquisite pleasure' by practising the following exercises in front of the bathroom mirror at least twice a day for a fortnight.

1 Pointing your tongue and pushing it forward a little, flicker it from side to side, keeping up a steady rhythm.
2 Still pointing, flicker it up and down, keeping up a steady rhythm.
3 With a broad tongue, practise lapping, with the focus on the upward movement of the tongue, therefore providing an upward beat.

ORAL MASSAGE

The Ray Stubbs massage school used to teach a number of amazing tongue strokes that can be used anywhere on the body but which especially resonate on the genitals. Ray Stubbs was a virtuoso massage teacher in the 1970s–1980s who has retired to sell books on the subject (See the appendix). Amongst his oral massage moves there are:

❧ Daisy Kisses. Plant small kisses, which contain just a little suction from your lips, all over your partner's body, including behind her knees and finishing off on the labia.

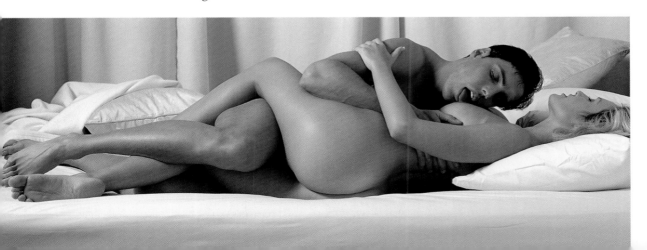

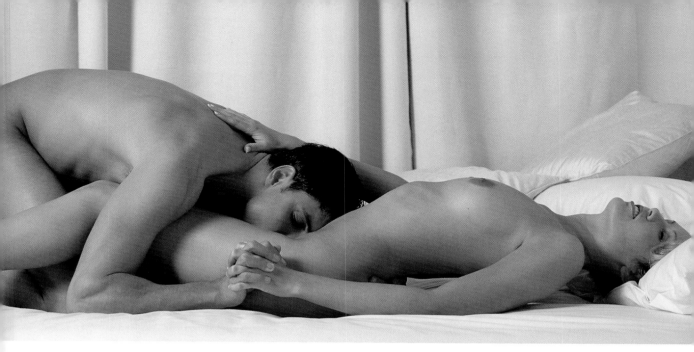

❦ Ice Cream Lick. Ray suggests treating your partner like a giant ice cream and, using the broad blade of your tongue, to lick her in luscious strokes.

❦ The Lipstick. Moistening part of her body and lavishly moistening your own lips, slide your lips gently backwards and forwards over the area as if you were applying lipstick.

❦ Snake Tongue. This is where your tongue twisters come in useful. Rapidly flicker the tip of your tongue across her flesh.

❦ School of Suction. Ray suggests gently sliding your lips, sucking on pathways along your partner's body. Gliding up the inner thigh can be effective because you meet her genitals at the top. You might try gently sucking at each of her labia. Then sliding up to the clitoris and sucking on this. You might continue to repeat the exercise, with the further option of flickering your tongue at the same time.

❦ In and Out Suction. Suck a nipple, or an earlobe or her clitoris gently into your mouth. Then while maintaining the suction, push with your tongue so that you are partially but not completely expelling the organ. Then draw the organ back in again. You can practise on your own fingertip to work out the best method. If you do this with an earlobe, be careful not to make sounds that will blast your loved one's eardrums.

TONGUE SEX

Ray always taught his special techniques as a wonderful form of massage but we believe that the movements he suggests are so appealing that it's probable your woman will turn them into something more aggressively sexual. Here are our suggestions to follow up:

- Always using the tip of the tongue in upward movement, lick from the entrance of the vagina up and over the clitoris repeatedly in short strokes.
- Try licking first to one side
- Then to the other
- Then over the top of the clitoris itself.
- Pointing the tongue, twirl it gently around the clitoris, first clockwise
- Then anti-clockwise.
- Then repeat the twirling actually on the vagina.
- Using the tip of the tongue, push gently and repeatedly on to one side of the clitoris.
- On to the other side
- On to the tip
- Combine gentle sucking with these strokes
- If one or more strokes prove especially effective, stay with these. Once something takes off erotically, women prefer repetition until they reach orgasm.

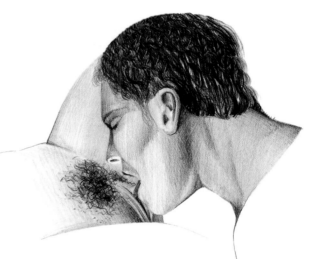

MEN'S MISTAKES

- The delicate bud of the clitoris is not as robust as the penis. Don't touch it too quickly or too hard.
- If you do not keep the area moist, the sensations turn from pleasure into pain.
- Don't use your tongue like a piston – more subtle strokes are needed.
- If you suck too hard, her genitals get desensitised.

ORAL SEX STATISTICS

When Alfred Kinsey formulated his famous sex reports in 1948, oral sex was hardly practised. All recent sex surveys show that it has been taken up with astonishing rapidity and is looked on today as commonplace. One survey showed in fact that many women have a greater desire for cunnilingus than their partners are apt to satisfy.

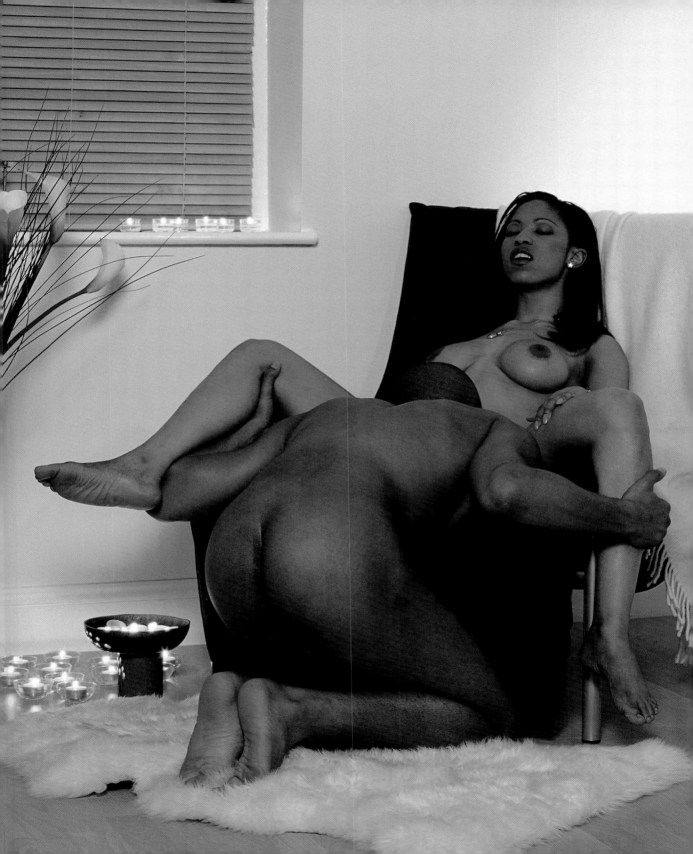

LOVE POSITIONS

It's clear by now that you are getting close to intercourse. But don't be limited by thinking good sex must include penetration. This is one of the myths of love-making. Good sex can be anything you desire. So don't worry if your woman explodes into climax without penetration. Don't feel left out if she subsides with a silly grin. Your turn will come, we promise.

Let us suppose that she has not yet climaxed and that she is begging you to stop that wonderful oral sex and 'come inside me – oh please'. Be aware that the changeover from direct clitoral stimulation to indirect genital stimulation will alter things. Unless she is so close to climaxing as makes no difference she will probably lose some of the benefits she's enjoyed so far.

If neither of you minds this, then intercourse can transport you to a newer and slower plane. If one of you however longs for orgasm to be soon and strong, the answer is to combine intercourse with finger stimulation. That way she gets direct *and* indirect clitoral stimulation all in one go. Here is how we would suggest you manage the dual combination.

UNDER YOUR THUMB

The reason why the missionary position proved so popular was that it proved the ideal sex position from which to worship the woman you love. Poised above her, and plunging into her, you are perfectly situated to feast visually on her flushed and passionate responses, to kiss as you thrust and to fondle her breasts as you push deeper into her. As a missionary you are in a position of power where you can depend on your masculine stamina to carry you on. You feel in control, you are in control, and if you want to bring your woman off quickly because you are none too certain you can maintain that control, your faithful right hand might slip right down, between your two bodies, and bring her prayers to a fit and fulfilling conclusion.

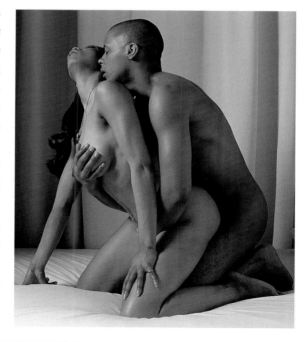

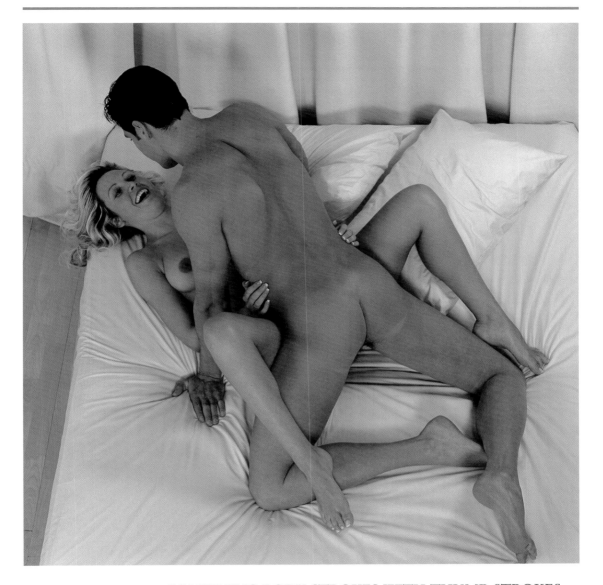

COMBINING BODY STROKES WITH THUMB STROKES

❦ To allow room for your hand to reach its objective and also to
give it some space in which to be dextrous, try experimenting in
your man-on-top position, so that you shift slightly to one side.

❦ Supporting yourself with one arm, reach down with the other so
that your hand locates her clitoris. You may find it necessary to sit
up slightly to make this possible and don't worry if it doesn't quite
work out to begin with. Practice makes perfect. At this angle, your

hand will feel as if it is the wrong way round, thus rendering it hard to offer her extra stimulation. This is why your thumb needs to be the perpetrator.

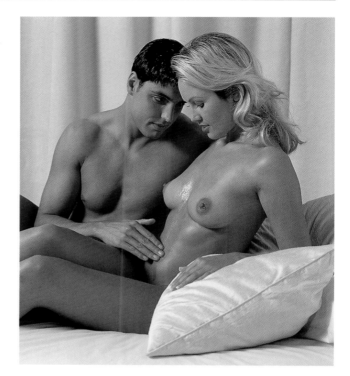

🌣 With your palm down and spread across her pubic mound, search gently with your thumb, for her clitoris. Your thumb needs to be slippery and your thumbnail short.

🌣 Having located the clitoris, stroke it gently and time the strokes so that they correspond with the thrusts your penis is making. For every surge of your penis, pull up with your thumb. On each occasion the penis is withdrawn, push down with the thumb. Make it so that the dual rhythm becomes absolutely synchronous. She is feeling two sets of stimulation in one.

🌣 Don't hit the clitoris too hard – you don't want to anaesthetize her. And constantly re-apply lubrication. The wetter, the slipperier, the hotter she gets, the better the sensation for her. Don't be disconcerted if her clitoris seems to disappear. It's there all right – keep searching and rubbing and whatever you do, keep up the rhythm. In fact, when the clitoris seems to disappear, this means that your woman is highly aroused. By this time, the rest of the spongy tissue around her pubis and the inner and outer labia are completely swollen with blood. Her genitals have reached the equivalent of a highly excited penis now bursting to express itself.

The versatile missionary position combines well with many other types of stimulation. If your lover is a woman who responds profoundly to breast stimulation (see the next chapter), caressing and rubbing the breasts while pulling your penis high up before rearing down into her again, becomes yet another wonderful option.

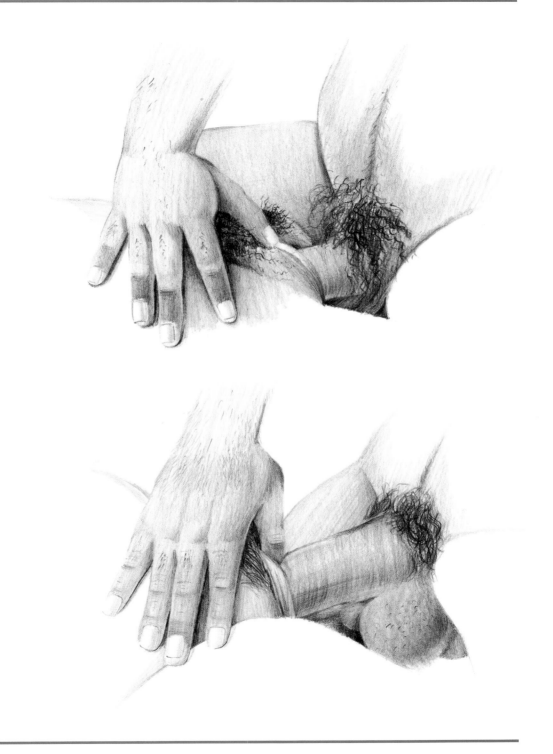

8 MORE ARTS OF good sex

There seems to be universal agreement that many men are attracted to breasts. Evolutionary theory would have it that breasts evolved to look like buttocks in order to encourage warmer and more direct intercourse between the human sexes. Be that as it may, there's an aspect of breast massage and breast stimulation that regularly gets left out of sex manuals. And this simple truth is that not *all* women like their breasts manipulated. Some women positively loathe the activity. If therefore your instinct is to make a dive for her cleavage, hold yourself in poised readiness but don't actually hurl yourself bosomwards.

Should you long to lose yourself in those globes, try patience. We believe that breast massage is a non-threatening method of finding out

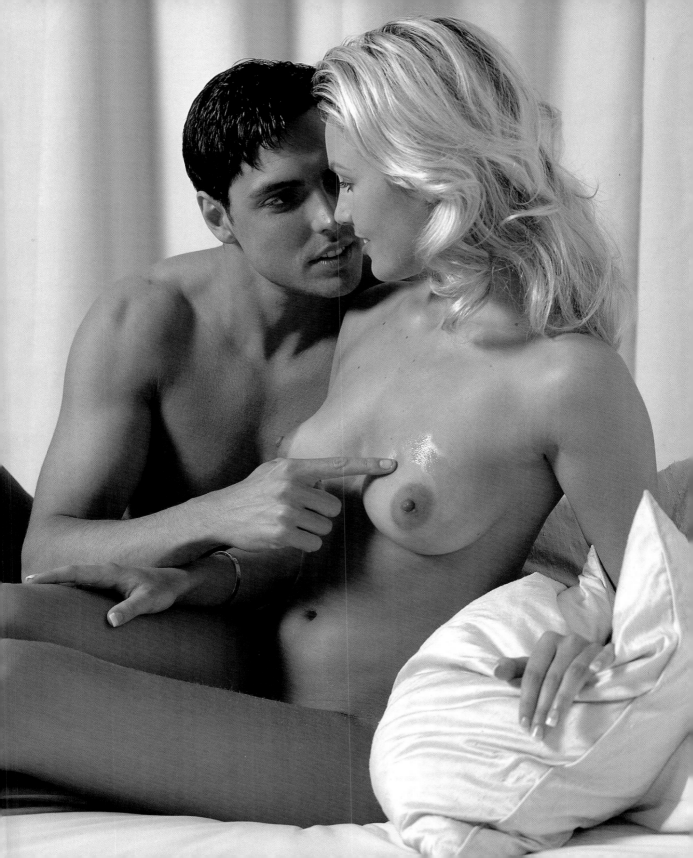

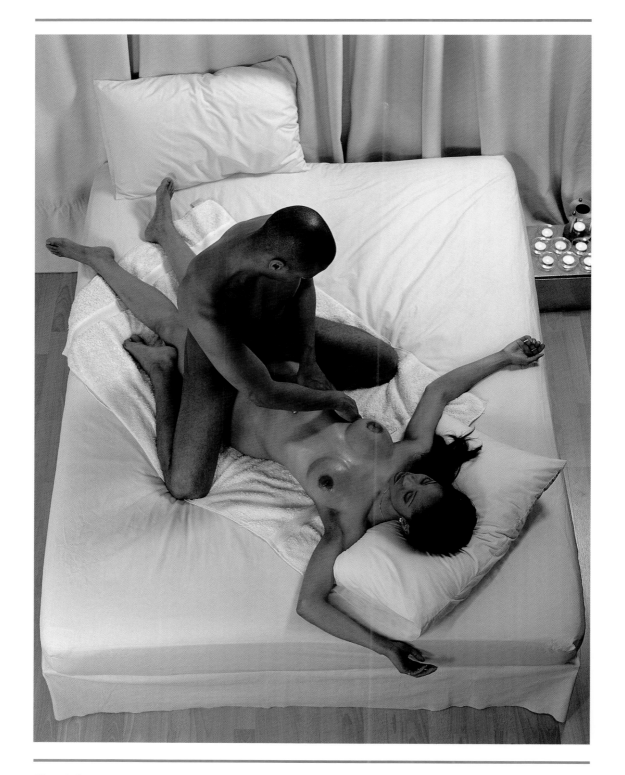

Masters and Johnson in their work comparing homosexual men, lesbian women and heterosexual couples, found that lesbians, during love-making:

❦ focused on the breasts. In some cases allotting as much as ten minutes of stimulation to each before moving on (and one stimulator climaxed simply from giving the stimulation!).

❦ The heterosexual control group, by contrast, were far less aroused whether giving or receiving.

whether your woman can actually stand to be touched there. You have to understand that breasts to some women are like the soles of the feet to many men – unbearably ticklish. It takes a confident handling for touch to become even remotely tolerable to such people. The upside of such over-sensitivity is that it often denotes someone with a particularly rapid sexual response.

TAKE IT EASY BREAST STROKES

For the benefit of breast men and responsive women we offer here our Take It Easy Breast Stroke Programme.

Offer warm sensual caresses on all parts of her body. As a matter of course, include the breasts in a slow and unhurried fashion. When she has settled down and relaxed to the treat you are offering, coat your hands lightly with a little warm massage oil and then begin.

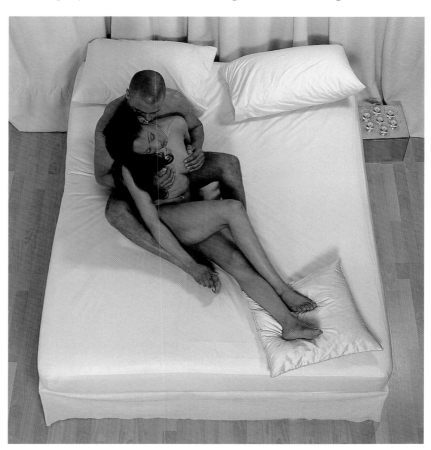

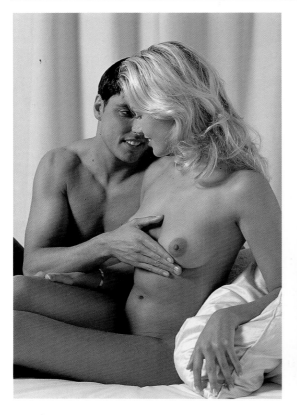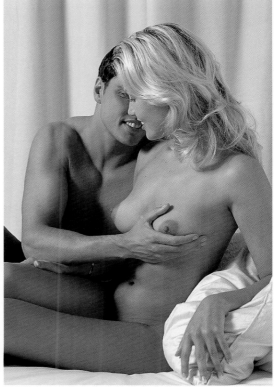

The Diagonals: Place your left hand just below and to the left of her left breast, palm downwards, your fingers pointing towards her right shoulder. Slowly and without pressure slide the flat of your hand up and over the left breast and diagonally off towards the right shoulder. Before your left hand ends the stroke, start another one in the same place with the right hand. The pattern therefore is hand-over-hand on the same diagonal for up to 10 strokes. Then do the same for the opposite diagonal. Because this is firm and predictable it does not sensually overload and most women can not only tolerate but actively enjoy it.

You can get a pretty good idea here of what she is going to find acceptable. What this particular stroke does is reassure. It allows her to feel confident that your touch will be bearable and by being non-threatening suggests that it might be wonderful to experience more. The greater relaxation she feels the greater toleration she will develop for your attention. Next you can graduate to something measurably more erotic.

The spirals: Coat a warm fingertip lightly with oil and (with fingernail well-trimmed,) gently and slowly circle the outside of her breast. On completing each lap, slightly shorten the circle a little so that your finger is effectively climbing a spiral around her breast, with the aim of ending at the tiny fixed point of the nipple, having circled it several times first. Experiment, during repetitions of the stroke, with different speeds and pressures and don't be afraid to ask which degree of firmness feels best.

The crab: With hands bunched in crab-like shapes, place them on a breast, fingertips only, either side of her nipple, and very slowly draw the hands apart and down the sides of the breast. Repeat for the other breast.

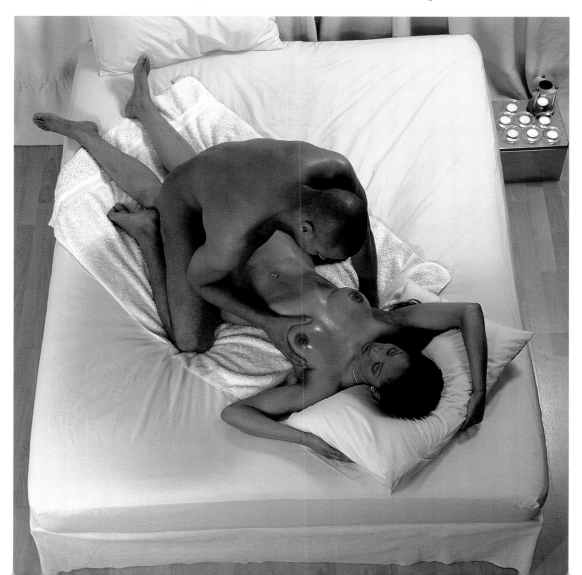

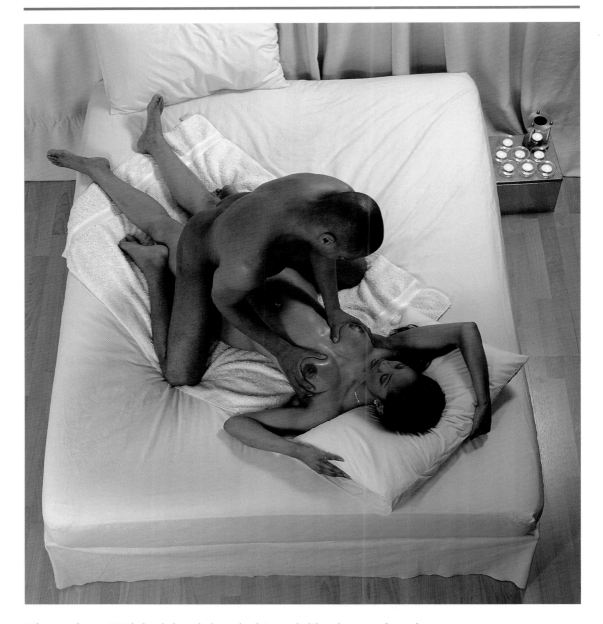

The seashore: With both hands bunched in crab-like shapes, place them on one breast, fingertips only, either side of her nipples and draw them down in opposite directions until they end diagonally apart, them draw them together again up and diagonally in the opposite direction. This constant together-then-apart motion is intended to feel like the tide going in and out at the seashore.

In order to be able to vary lovemaking with our partner, it helps to know if we can vary it with ourselves. The more we learn to respond to new stimuli the more ability we gain to expand our sensual options and avoid getting in a rut. One suggestion is for you and your lover to take it in turns at very lightly stroking the area around the genitals and then the genitals themselves, with a touch like a feather. You might even try using a feather. Vary the direction and the length of the strokes. You aren't aiming at an orgasm – just to discover what sensation this arouses and let your partner know. Include the perineum and don't forget the anus.

Lift off: As a finale, try lightly squeezing a nipple between finger and thumb and then sliding up and off only to be replaced by the other hand doing the same thing until you have set up a regular motion.

Always repeat breast massage on the other breast. Always keep things slow, lubricated and warm. Stop if she ever looks uncomfortable.

STROKING ALL OVER

Most of the moves we've suggested so far have depended on the skills of touch. When Masters and Johnson carried out their pioneering work comparing the love-making patterns of gays and heterosexuals, they realised what heterosexuals could learn from the gays. While heterosexual men and women aimed at orgasm spending relatively little time on the rest of the body, homosexual lovers spent ages stimulating and stroking each other all over with the ultimate result of a supercharged sexual response. One of the regular complaints of straight men and women seeking coun-selling is that somehow sex doesn't feel entirely satisfactory *so this may well be because they are overlooking the value of total tactile stimulation.*

Please note, so far we've rationed use of the dreaded word 'fore-play'. This is because the word is such a misnomer. Foreplay makes body caresses sound as if they are only a minor preliminary to the real enjoy-ment of sex. In fact, foreplay *is* to a large extent sex and since touch is such an integral element of this book we are not going to list a special foreplay section here – touch suggestions and touch exercises are scat-tered throughout.

SEXERCISE – EXTRA STIMULATION

Bodies possess many sensitive areas, all of which long for extra stimulation during intercourse. Something additional and dynamic can often be added. We've talked about combining stimulating her clitoris while making love in the man-on-top position. Another useful exercise is to:

- Talk with your partner about the areas she might specifically like to receive more sensual attention.

- Then to work out an intercourse position that allows you easier access to these parts of the body.

- Then spend a good 20 minutes experimenting with such positions.

CLITORAL STIMULATION

Every woman masturbates in a way that is uniquely and individually her own. Some women stimulate the whole of their genital area; this method usually takes longer for climax but reputedly causes stronger and more satisfying orgasms than by clitoral touching alone and is unlikely to be painful or irritating. Other women however concentrate mainly on the clitoris. (There is a small percentage of women who come into a first relationship having never masturbated at all. They expect to find out about their bodies from their experience with their lover.)

GETTING TO KNOW HER

If you want to offer your woman manual stimulation – and as a wonderful lover you surely do – you might, as you practise your strokes on her genitals, ask her casually the following questions:

- ❦ Does she like to be stroked all over the genitals?
- ❦ Does she prefer touch on one side or the other of the labia?
- ❦ Does she prefer touch on one side or the other of the clitoris?

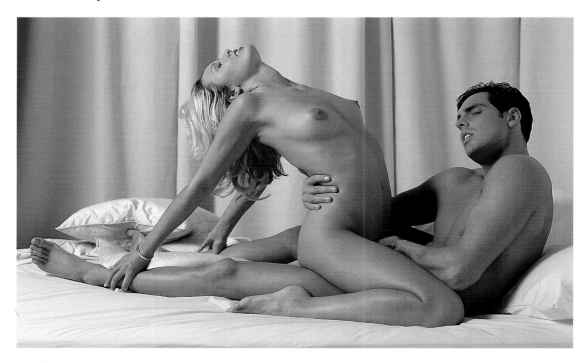

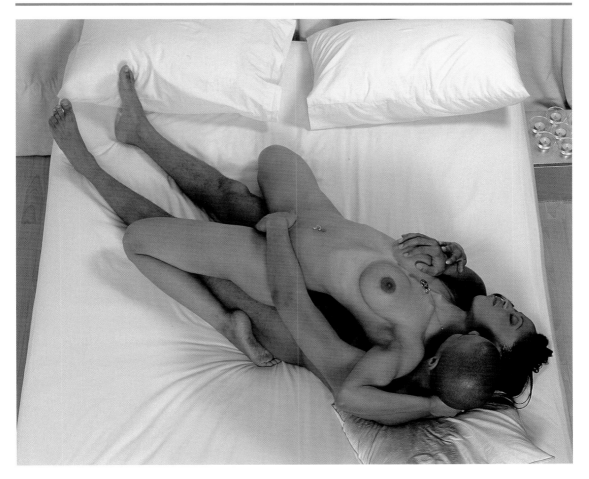

- How does she feel about her anus being touched?
- Does she like her clitoris specifically stimulated?
- Or would she prefer indirect stimulation?
- Does she like or dislike finger penetration during genital stimulation?
- If she does like it, does she prefer your finger to simply rest inside her or to thrust?

We're not suggesting you subject her to a rigorous cross-examination – just that as the two of you enjoy yourselves you might drop the occasional relevant question into the proceedings.

Many of the patterns described in the oral sex section in the previous chapter can be re-applied when making love to your woman by loving touch. What follows here are some suggestions for how genital and clitoral stimulation might go. But it is up to you to find out her very own specific pattern of erotic response. Don't be frightened to ask, even to suggest that she might demonstrate some of her preferred masturbation strokes. Some sex therapy methods teach the woman to put her finger over her partner's finger and guide it so that she effectively teaches him how to stimulate her.

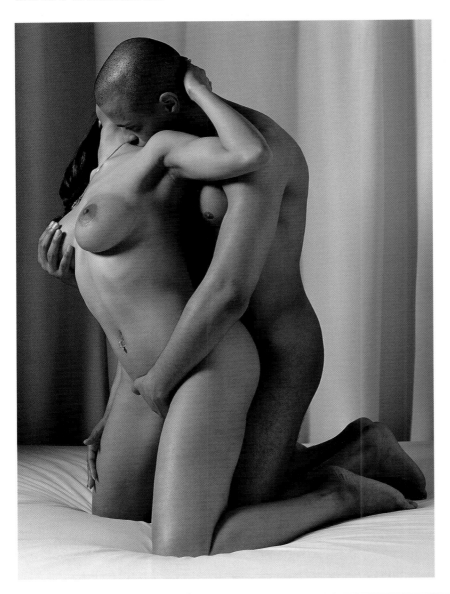

The lesbian women studied
by Masters and Johnson
shared a dislike with many
heterosexual women, of
deep finger penetration and
rarely did it to each other.
Those women who have
active G-spot sensation may
like two- or three-finger
pressure on the front wall of
the vagina but usually only
after they are already highly
aroused.

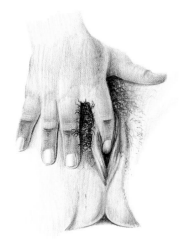

CLITORAL STIMULATION

The first golden rule is to ensure that your lover's genitals are moist before massaging or caressing. If she needs extra moisture, use massage oil or saliva. The second golden rule is that genital stimulation needs to come long after the rest of the body has been primped and pampered.

❦ Lying to one side of your partner, stretch your hand across and lightly rub and stroke the insides of her thighs, bringing your hand towards her genitals each time and brushing them lightly before going back towards the knee again.

❦ Bring the genitals more specifically into the picture by brushing with your whole hand, up across her labia towards the pubic mound. Do not be rough, make these moves slowly and deliberately linger.

❦ On about the third whole hand movement upwards, let one of your fingers 'accidentally' glance inside the labia so that it skims the entrance to the vagina and brushes inside the pubic area, bumping against the clitoris on the way up. Repeat this two or three times.

❦ Focusing your finger more specifically, pull it up against the underside of the clitoris and let it bump across the top surface of the clitoris.

❦ Using a highly lubricated forefinger only, delicately saw at one side of the clitoris, up and down.

❦ Do the same on the other side of the clitoris.

❦ Gently rim around the clitoris with a fingertip (short fingernails only).

❦ Gently rim in the opposite direction. These strokes can be done with the main part of the finger held away from the clitoris, then with the main part of the finger right up against the clitoris.

❦ Circle directly on the clitoris, so lightly that you are barely touching.

Of course there are many other ways in which to give your woman a wonderful genital experience but these are some of the basics. Enjoy compiling your own directory.

LOVE'S CLEANING LADY

We've left it a bit late here to talk about the setting in which you make love. But even the appearance of your bedroom makes an impact on your woman's psyche. If it is clean and tidy and sweet smelling, with candle flames dancing and warmth filtering through the air, this will create a sensual impression. If, on the other hand, the room is a tip, smells of old socks, there's half a sandwich on the edge of the bed and a bright pink sex toy down the side, she is going to feel extremely uncomfortable. So think seriously about whether or not you intend to bring your lover back to it. And if you do, clear up and clean up.

CHARMER SUTRA

(Yhe sexual art of love positions most likely to bring tears of joy – not pain – to your lover's eyes) There are probably as many love-making positions as there are nights in the year. And almost as many editions of the *Kama Sutra* to illustrate the point. We aim to invent here our very own version of the lovers' classic, only with one major advantage. We include only those positions that will specifically stimulate your woman. (See the companion volume to this book *How to Make Great Love to a Man* to find the male equivalents).

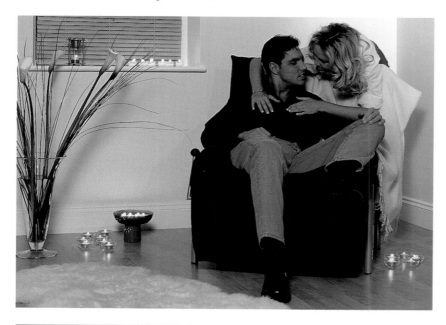

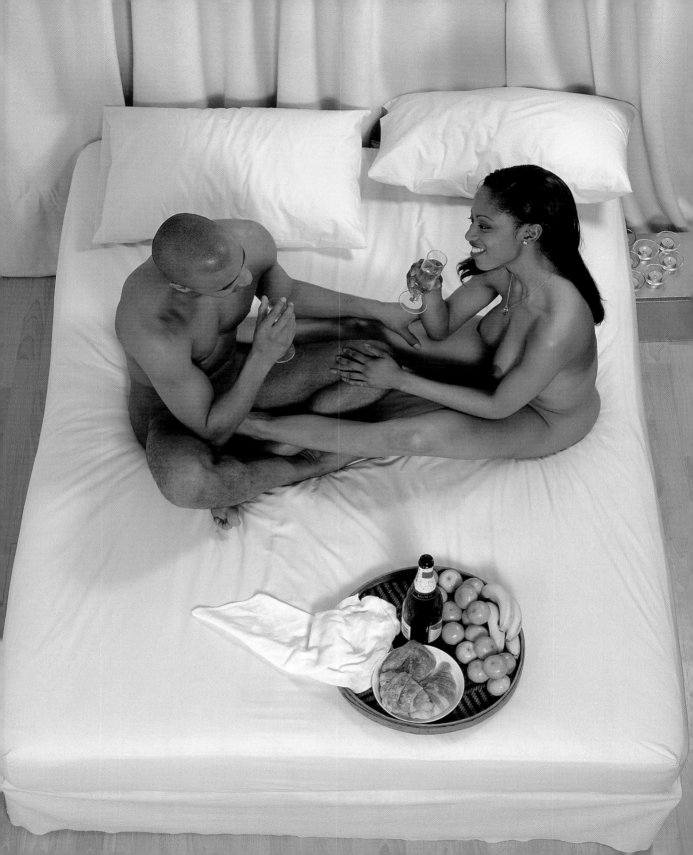

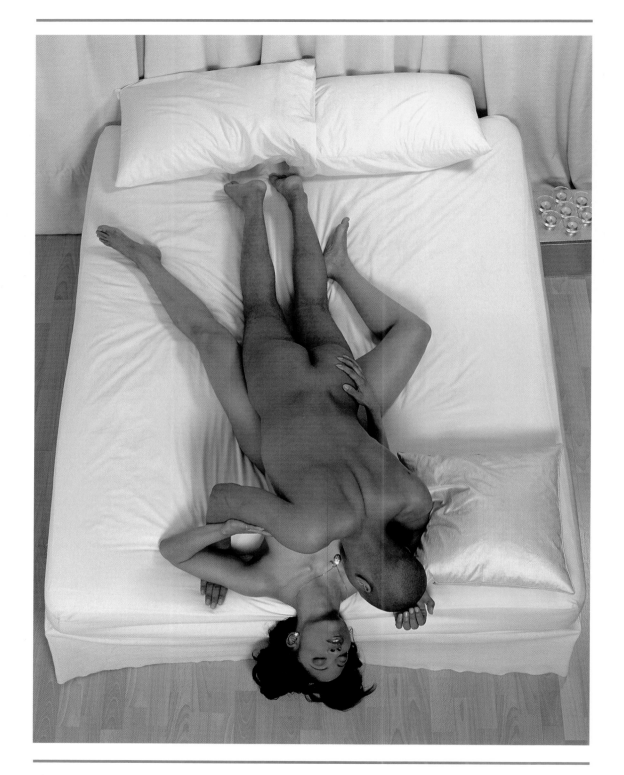

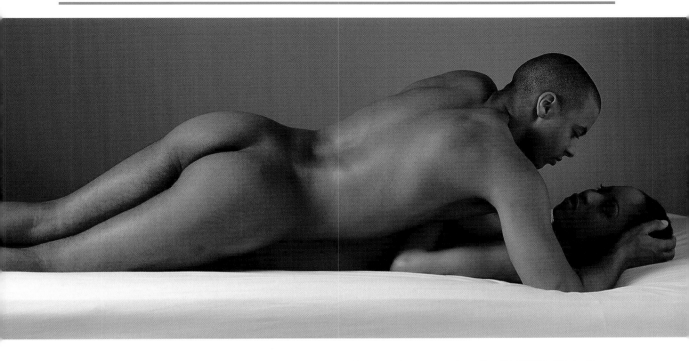

THE MISSIONARY POSITION

We've already waxed lyrical about the Missionary Position in the previous chapter. It is by far the most common sex position in European and American cultures. As recently as 1948, Alfred Kinsey discovered that 70 per cent of Americans had never had sex in any other way. Since then later surveys have indicated that we are more likely to vary love positions depending on the level of education we have received. If you are college educated for example, you are more likely to use a variety of love positions than if you left school early and went out to work. However, the missionary still ranks high.

This face-to-face, man-on-top position offers the opportunity to kiss, caress and watch each other's faces during sex. It's relatively easy to achieve and is best started off with the woman opening her legs apart, with her knees bent. If you encounter any difficulty guiding your penis into her vagina she is well positioned to reach down with a hand and to help. So too are you. The beauty of the missionary is that it allows you to balance on both knees and one arm, thus freeing up the second arm for all manner of amicable activity.

SIXTEEN TONS AND WHAT DO YOU GET?

One of the problems of heavier men is their belief that their woman constitutes a curvaceous style of mattress. Not so. If you allow your weight to collapse upon your woman at any stage of the proceedings, including the fateful time after you have had your orgasm, you stand a good chance of squashing her. One of the benefits of the missionary is that you can support yourself with your limbs and prevent her from being crushed.

Another benefit is that most women are less strong than men. Should they get the opportunity to be on top, they may find it hard to continue because of the puff factor. Also, being rather more passive suits some weaker members of the sex. Since this makes you the one with the real range of movement it becomes necessary to remind you that she may need encouragement to shift around beneath you. This is especially important if she really gets off on deep thrusting.

KNEES UP AND BOOMPS A DAISY

The subtle adjustment of helping her to pull her knees up and back during the missionary position is one way of assisting her to deeper penetration. If she doesn't know whether or not this is good for her, take such powerful strokes extremely easily. Some women possess an over-sensitive cervix at the end of the vagina and slamming in to it can shock and bruise, not tempt and delight. There are however individuals whose cervical area is very sensitive to deep thrusting and who find that its stimulation sends up erotic responses to the whole of the body.

THE C-SPOT

One of the great mysteries of male and female sexual fit is that there appears to be a design fault. The penis penetrates the vagina neatly enough but unfortunately never directly touches the C-Spot (the clitoris). Unless … slight adjustments are made during the missionary position. One of these adjustments is for you to snuggle hard up against her pubic mound penetrating her deeply, but not thrusting. Instead, you make very slight rocking movements against her pubic mound. If you have managed to angle yourself slightly up and over her pubic mound, there's a high likelihood that the shaft of your penis will reach direct contact with your lover's C-Spot and that your pelvic rocking now offers

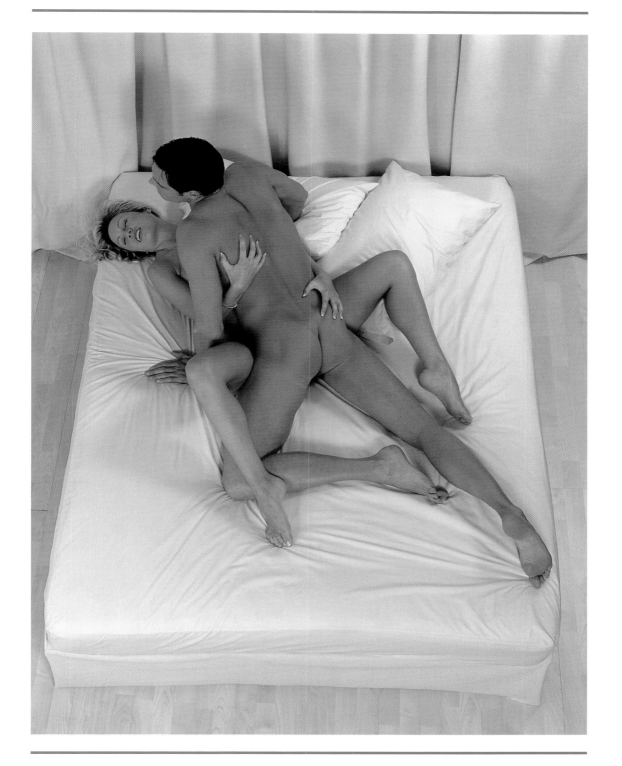

direct and persistent stimulation without bruising or anaesthetising. This subtle form of deep penetration during the missionary position may offer a very easy route to your woman's orgasm.

THE G-SPOT

The Grafenberg Spot, known popularly as the G-Spot, is named after the German gynaecologist Ernst Grafenberg. It's described as a pressure-sensitive area on the anterior wall of the vagina. When pressed in the right way it triggers orgasm. Not every woman however appears to have such a spot and there is a lot of debate about whether or not it actually exists. One Israeli researcher Dr Zwei Hock carried out a six-year study of the female genitalia and found that the *entire area* of the anterior wall of the vagina, rather than one particular area, is richly endowed with sexual nerve endings.

Which brings us back to the missionary position. Anterior wall in this case refers to the upper wall of the vagina, the interior section snuggled underneath the pubis. It does not refer to the ground floor, the lower section of the vaginal canal that lies next to the perineum or pelvic floor. If you think about the geometry of penetration it doesn't take advanced calculation to get a vision of the penis pushing (at least partially) into that anterior wall during missionary position sex. Hence another good reason to suggest that your woman might like to put her knees up and back.

THE STRAITJACKET

Another variation on the missionary is the legs-straight-out-in-front once intercourse has begun. If your woman has specially sensitive outer lips (labia) this position offers an intense method of holding the lips bunched firmly against the penis so that they gain maximum stimulation.

WOMAN ON TOP

This position probably comes second in the popularity stakes. A 1974 survey showed it to be used by nearly three-quarters of all married couples at least occasionally. Sometimes the woman just wants to initiate sex and sliding neatly on top of the erect penis that she has just coaxed into life is an excellent method of doing so. Another time-honoured method of reaching the woman-on-top position is the Swiss Roll. Here, although intercourse is started off in the missionary position, one or other of the participants gives a mighty heave and the couple rolls over, reversing their polarities.

The advantages of woman-on-top are many. It allows her to be an active participant and to retain a sense of control. It means that she can regulate the tempo, the movements and the depths of penetration. It's no accident that sex therapy methods particularly use this position on the

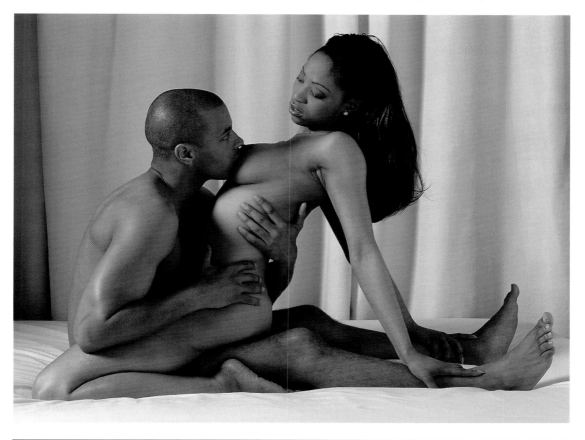

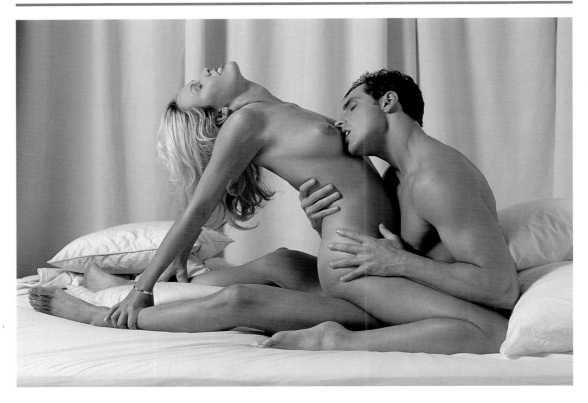

grounds that many women can arrange the angle of thrusting so that their clitoris is in the direct firing line and therefore stands the maximum chance of being pleasured.

Points for you to notice – as you lie there, taking things easy, you can let your hands wander. You can stroke and caress her buttocks, her torso and her breasts. You can offer her a variety of massage while she labours over you. And of course, because the two of you are face-to-face, you can keep in touch with every fleeting expression and thus gauge her feelings and reactions.

Beware: Don't assume that every woman enjoys this position. Some women feel very exposed up there on top, getting the sense that they are being watched. Others, who react passively, feel adrift. They don't really know what to do nor do they feel confident enough to experiment.

Beware: Don't let your penis slip out, which can happen easily in this position. Be prepared to help it back into place.

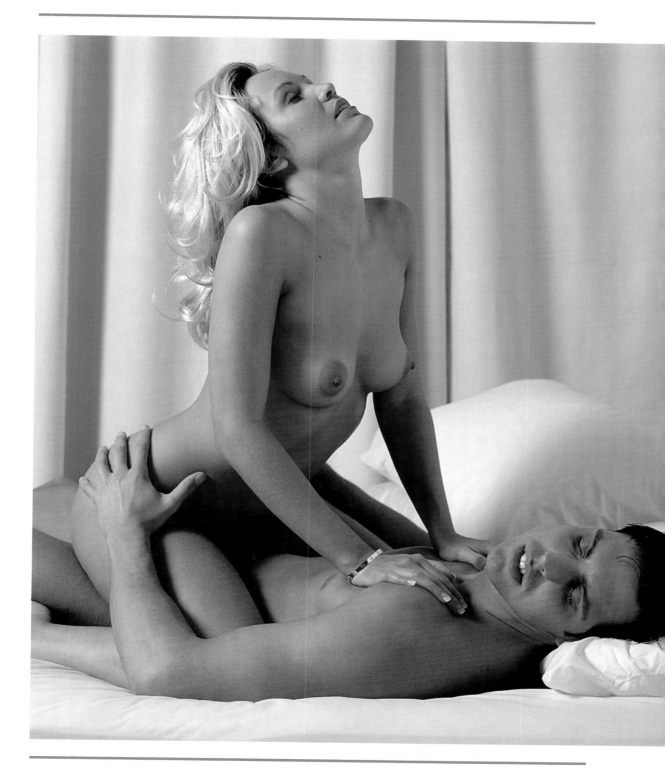

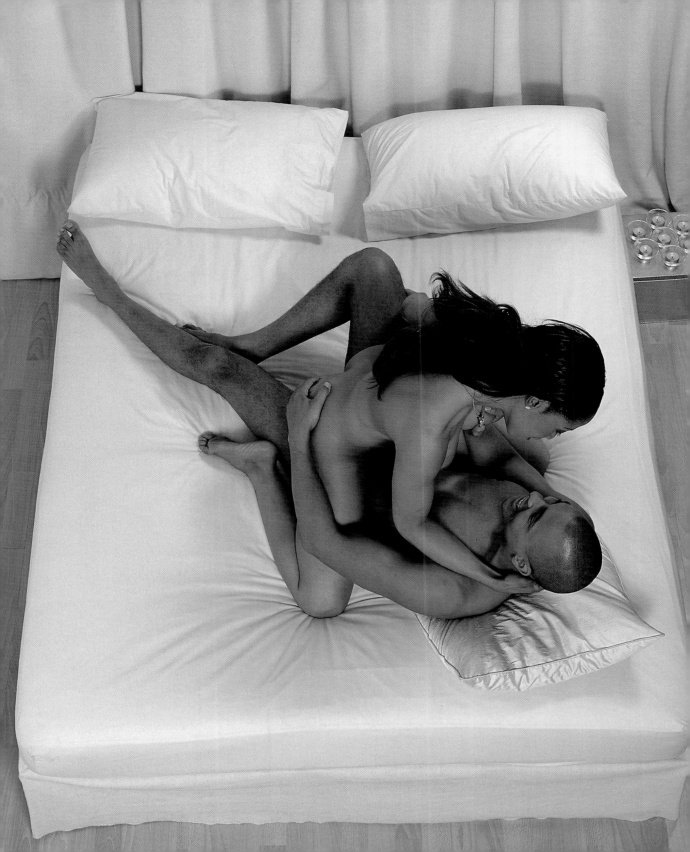

WOMAN-ON-TOP VARIATIONS

The easiest way for her to manage this position is by leaning down along your body so that your faces are within kissing distance. This feels loving and affectionate and prevents her from feeling high up and exposed. But it is a position that puts a lot of strain on her strength. She needs powerful muscles to continue to prop herself up by the arms for any length of time. She also needs a flexible spine and strong buttock and leg muscles to continue without flaking out exhausted.

If she doesn't possess these attributes, she might prefer the sitting upright version of the woman-on-top. This is less tiring but will not unfortunately give her much clitoral stimulation since the upright seat takes her clitoris away from any direct contact. This is where a thumbs-on extra move can give her the incentive to continue. Using either of your thumbs, tuck them underneath her so that at least one meets with the clitoris and rubs with a rhythm to match the tempo she is keeping up with you.

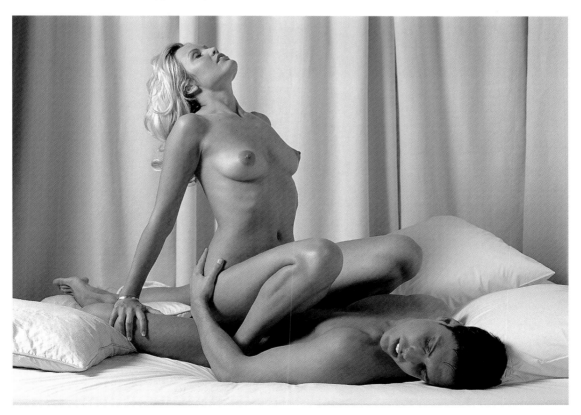

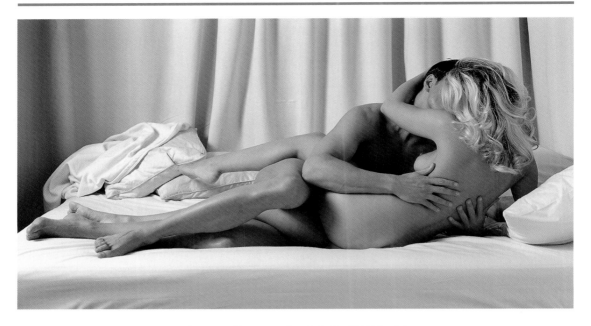

FACE TO FACE, SIDE BY SIDE

Sounds like the title of a song and if it were so, it would need to be one
with a slow, relaxed beat. If you want your woman to feel a strong sense
of friendship, if you would like her to think of you as an affectionate
man who enjoys spending time on her and with her, this is a good position. It won't do a lot for your climaxes but as a gorgeous friendship
activity, it's great.

The chief advantage is that neither partner is pinned down by the
weight of the other so problems of fatigue and muscle cramps are elim-
inated. Both partners are free to control pelvic thrusting. If you are a lot
taller than your woman a version that allows the woman to effectively
wrap herself around you, while supported, at the same time, by your
arms, is invaluable.

There are several ways of doing this but the one that allows you
most mobility is where you face each other lying on your sides and
where you lift your woman's upper leg over your top thigh, tucking her
lower leg into place between your thighs. With an arm slipped underneath her, partially raise her off the ground so that she closely faces
you. Your arm acts as a fulcrum or pivot so that every time she shifts
away from you, you can push her back towards you as you thrust.

Steve told us that 'I used to wake up feeling horny, in the middle of the night and slip inside my girlfriend in the spoons position. She would wake up halfway through arousal, (her arousal) and would be so relaxed from sleep that her orgasm would take her by surprise. On more than one occasion, she told me she had been dreaming about having sex and then woke up to find that she was.

'There was one night when she turned the tables on me. I woke up to find that she had wriggled her buttocks over my cock which she had stimulated by hand and had actually slipped herself over and on to it and she was well on the way to climaxing by the time I woke up. I'm a very heavy sleeper and she told me afterwards, she had been doing this for at least 20 minutes. I was just sorry to have missed out on things.'

SPOONING

Snuggle up to your woman's back and tuck her closely into the contours of your body. If you wriggle around her buttocks you can place your penis firmly between her thighs and partially penetrate her vagina. There is something lazily relaxed about this; it's the kind of love position suited to a warm night, a roaring log fire and a cosy cuddle between the sheets. Some women are so turned on by sex from the rear that they can climax without any additional stimulation. Most women however prefer a little extra. The beauty of this snuggle is that your upper hand is positioned to creep around her thighs and stroke her relaxedly between the legs. It's a good position from which to begin intercourse after sleeping.

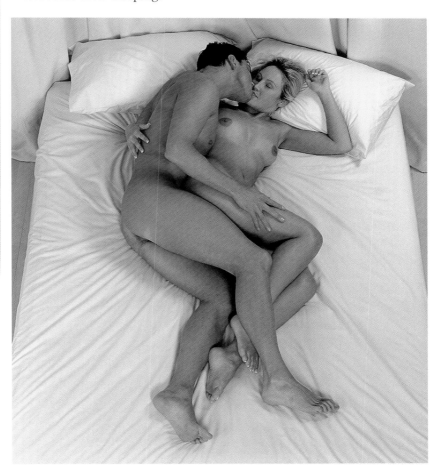

REAR ENTRY – DOGGY STYLE

Probably the most comfortable of several different ways of doing this rear entry position is with your woman kneeling on the floor with her upper half resting on the bed and you kneeling behind her. Very few women can climax directly from rear entry sex so for her to gain maximum sensation you need to stretch out a hand and (reaching around her thigh) find her clitoris with your fingertip. However, the fact that her thighs are resting up against the side of the bed means that it may be difficult for your hand to get much mobility. The alternative position, doggy-style on the bed, where she rests her arms and shoulders on the bed but sticks her rear into the air, means that she can steady herself against your thrusting while allowing plenty of space in which to manoeuvre your hands and fingers.

Many women find the animalistic style of this position extremely exciting because it's associated with 'forbidden' sex. But the fact that her buttocks can be spread wide, thus additionally exposing the anus, is also a source of excitement. People often don't know that the outside edge of the anus is rimmed with rich nerve endings and that contact with this area can be highly arousing.

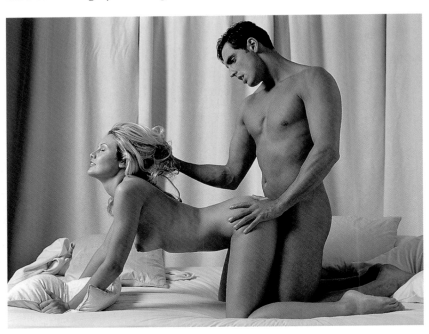

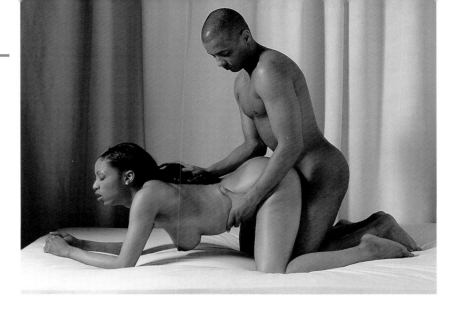

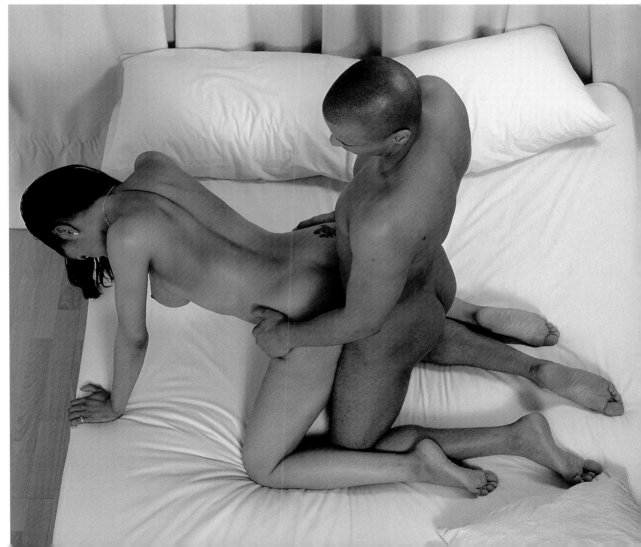

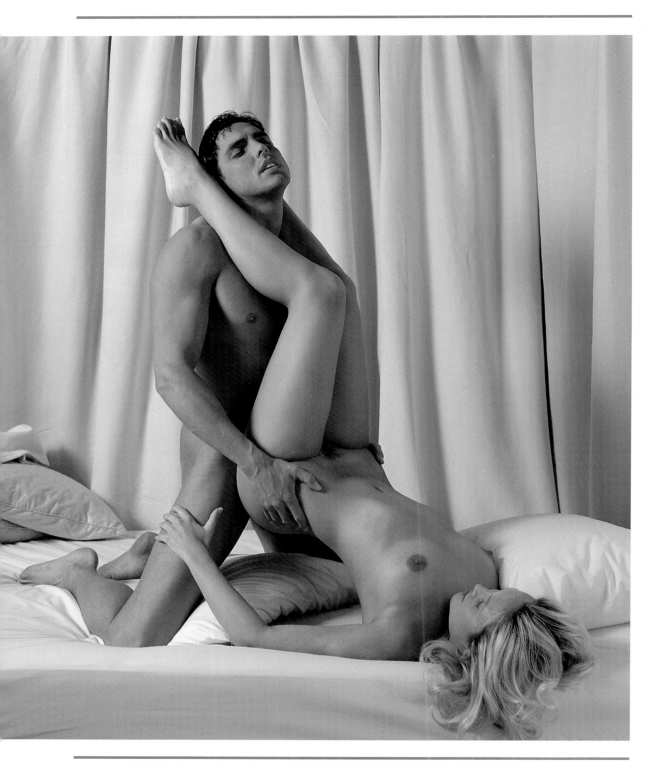

SPECIALIST SHOTS

THE SCISSORS

This is a particularly useful position if you are very heavy or if your partner is pregnant. In either case, of course, you don't want to squash her. This position is so named because, looked on from above, the man's head and shoulders naturally rest to the side of his partner's and the couple forms a scissors shape. Using your abdomen on top of hers to form a type of fulcrum, put one knee between her legs and the other outside her legs so that you are effectively trapping one of her legs. Her other (free) leg can bend back and up allowing you to penetrate still quite deep. Your upper body lies above and to one side of her. The big advantage as far as she is concerned is that you can press up against her genitals with the whole of the top of your thigh giving her clitoris intense sensation.

G-SPOT SPECIAL

This is particularly effective for caressing the anterior wall of the vagina although it is not so good for making contact with the clitoris. Here the woman lies on her back. You kneel up and clasping her buttocks draw her forwards so that her buttocks are resting on your thighs, near enough for you to penetrate her vagina. If, having inserted your penis inside, you then lean back a little, the angle of the penis rises up hard against that upper vaginal wall. Small rocking movements and concentrated pressure if continued for a time can be enough to trigger her to orgasm.

ACROBATIC ADVENTURES

LEGS UP

There are many love positions that do not offer much direct clitoral stimulation but which are nevertheless exciting because they feel especially erotic. One of those is where she is lying on her back with her legs high in the air and he is penetrating her missionary style but with her legs actually resting on his shoulders. You might coax her into this position by slipping one of your arms under one of her knees and helping that leg up, then doing the same with the other leg.

DOING THE SPLITS

A variation of the above is where you help her raise one leg up over your shoulder and then press with your other hand on her other leg so that it is lying out completely flat to one side of your legs. She is effectively doing the splits while lying on her back. This varies the sensation that she experiences and because her inner thigh muscles are being stretched, allows her to feel extremely sensuous. You do need to feel confident however that she is reasonably supple otherwise you might instead provoke cries of agony.

DOING THE FROG

One of the risks that people writing sex manuals take is of getting far too serious. This is a pity because the best sex is fun. It's fun fooling around, finding that the two of you trust each other enough to become silly infants again. It's fun, collapsing with giggles at having just tried an advanced and impossible position. This is why we enjoy including mention of The Frog. In this woman-on-top position, she lies above you with her feet propped up on yours, thus giving herself purchase. Your own legs are splayed so that hers must be too. This means that you both feel your genitals are partially exposed. In order to rise and fall in the action of thrusting, your woman now needs to push off with her feet. In order to do so, you need to make sure your feet resist the pressure, rather than giving way so that she collapses. It sounds pretty silly; it *is* pretty silly. But it's a great laugh if you're in a fun mood.

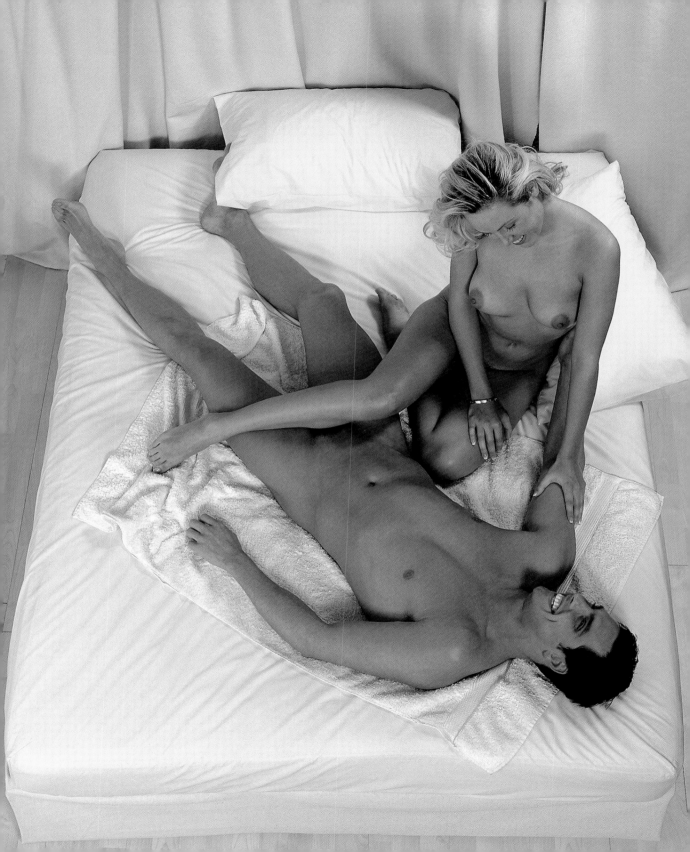

UP AGAINST THE FURNITURE

HALF ON, HALF OFF

This position is one where the woman lies on her back on the bed but with her legs dangling over the side and her feet on the floor. The man kneels up between her legs so that his penis is right-angled towards her vagina. This is another position that favours the G-spot but there's also something free and abandoned about making love while virtually slipping off the bed. This is a position that offers erotic inspiration even though it does little for her climax. Since she is so well supported by the bed you can bring a free hand into play in the direction of her clitoris and make up for any deficiencies of thrust.

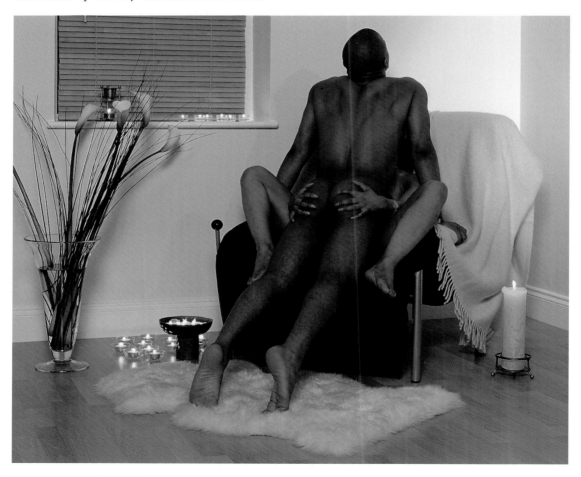

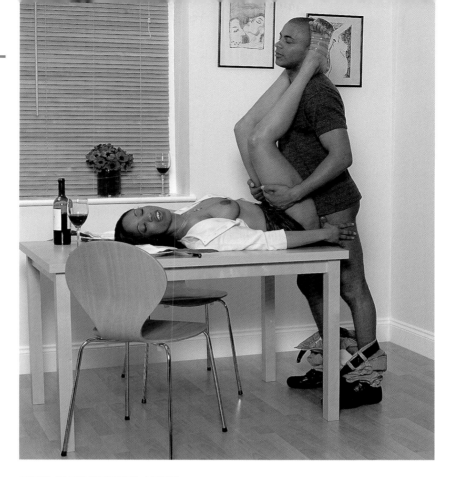

THE DOMESTIC ARTS

Another version of the above is where the woman lies on the kitchen table with her legs dangling over the side. Since she is unlikely here to be able to rest her feet on the ground it means that you have to hold on to her buttocks pretty firmly as you pull her towards you during thrusting. You meanwhile are standing up, probably with your legs slightly bent, so that your penis can be angled to table top and vagina level. This is a position for temporary fun only, since it will do little for your mate's arousal and may prove uncomfortable because table tops are hard to lie on. Why do it? Because it brings variety into play and novelty is an important factor when establishing and continuing a love life. But there is another reason. It's what we call the up-against-the-living-room-wall factor. There are times when you are so hot for each other and so urgently desirous of tearing the clothes off each other's back in order to fuck, that actually doing so in uncomfortable circumstances adds to the excitement and positively enhances arousal.

UP AGAINST THE LIVING-ROOM WALL

This form of intercourse is associated with the urgency of early sexual attraction and takes on an especially intense eroticism all of its own. We don't recommend resorting to it in the very first instances of having sex. That's because it's too rapid, too urgent, can be almost violent. This is wonderful when you already know that sex between you is amazing and a rare intimacy is evolving. But it could be potentially disturbing during earlier days when none of these things are yet established.

This sex position is pretty self-evident but for the sake of those who have never experienced its actuality, here's how:

❦ Lean your woman with her back to the wall with her legs slightly apart. Support her at the rear with one hand while helping to insert your penis with the other. If she is short, you may have to lift her slightly. You may also have to bend your legs so that your penis is suitably angled. Don't forget that every time you thrust you crash her into the wall – so do your best to partly cushion her back with a free hand. This is exciting as long as your woman is shorter than you. Because of the height difference, you cannot help thrusting upwards and if you press in close your penis should be able to rub and thrust near or possibly on her clitoris. But the position's strongest advantage is that it reeks of excitement, urgency and lust. It can be a massive turn-on in itself.

The Perfumed Garden offers some extremely useful variations of the upright position, including the powerfully athletic Driving the Peg Home, where the male actually lifts the female off the ground until her vagina is at right angles to his upright penis and her knees grasp his thighs as if she were riding a horse. There is also a See-Saw version where the woman hitches one leg over her partner's thigh, thus offering a wider and more comfortable stimulation, and where the couple are exhorted to take it in turns to thrust, first one, then the other, a kind of alternative in-and-out so that each partner gains a sense of control and a choice of angle.

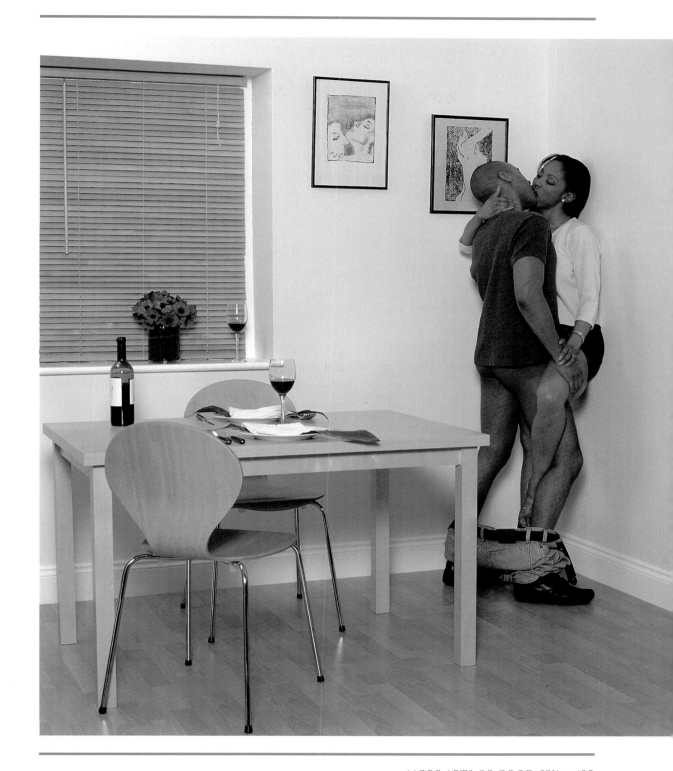

THE ART STUDENT'S SEX MANUAL

Finally there is a range of sex positions outlined in the ancient *Tao of Sex* that appear to be performed purely for their artistic appearance. We suggest carrying out a few of these in front of a remote-controlled camera so that you might later enjoy the photos as an additional and creative turn-on. You might consider:

SWALLOWS IN LOVE

In this man-on-top position, the man lies with his legs straight out behind him while she extends her straight legs at a slight angle to him so that the couple takes on the v-shaped tail of the swallow. She meanwhile grasps his waist with both hands while he lies over her kissing her neck.

TWO FISHES

In this side-by-side intercourse each partner lies with legs stretched down, top leg resting on the lower one. He helps her raise her legs off the ground by holding her thighs with the hand he is not leaning on, so that her thighs rest across his. Viewed from the side the couple looks like a pair of fish waving their tails relaxedly around each other.

BUTTERFLIES IN FLIGHT

This is a woman-on-top variation where the couple lies with their feet straight out and where she rests her toes on his feet and pushes herself up off from his toes. Once intercourse has begun, both partners hold hands and stretch out their arms to the side. As she pushes off with her feet she rears her head and then lowers it on relaxation. The overall effect is like the slow flapping of butterfly wings.

All suggestions about love positions are merely ... suggestions. We hope to offer you inspiration but we certainly do not wish to pressure or dictate. Spontaneous sex is exciting but even when it leaps up out of nowhere, taking you by surprise, *how* it actually happens is still contingent on how much you know. We hope we have paid some useful information into your memory banks!

THE MR D'ARCY
factor
(USING EROTIC NARRATIVE)

Research on sexual fantasy shows that far more men get turned on by fantasy material than do women. Women have difficulty in recognising that they even respond to stimulating films or books, and sometimes deny their arousal. And yet they *are* aroused. Studies in the laboratory, where women are wired to machines monitoring physiological response, prove this conclusively.

We offer the suggestion that men and women get turned on by *different things*. Men respond to sexy photographs and high-action written erotica. Women get excited by a very different type of reading material that most men would not categorise as sexy at all. The enormous success of Mills and Boon novels bears witness to the fact that women are highly stimulated by reading about mood and romance. It's the Mr D'Arcy factor, the powerful legs encased in skin-tight breeches, the tall shiny riding boots, the thought of those massive thighs gripping the glistening, sweaty flanks of the stallion, that excites. The eroticism lies in the power of suggestion, the choice of words, the plain *lack* of anything overtly sexual, the fact that this is safely classified as romance and can therefore be experienced as non-threatening. Many men would have a hard time getting through the books in the first place, let alone seeing what was so titillating about them.

Many little girls grow up reading emotive literature, or watching or listening to it. They get to associate first arousal with dramatic action in the stories. When the heroines swoon, they feel the passions. They learn to associate such swooning, that wonderful helpless absorbing sexy feeling, with the power of men being masterful. And so, entire generations of women learn to respond to sexy narratives. Of course this is not directly admitted, even to themselves, since acknowledgement might place the activity out of bounds. Turning on via Barbara Cartland is so alien to the male experience (of turning on via handling their genitals and thinking of a supermodel in thigh boots) that most men, including male sex researchers, don't even know the phenomenon exists.

Incidentally, laboratory studies have shown that women don't *only* get turned on by the softer stuff. They get turned on by blue films, and bluer reading material as well – it's just that once again, they don't always recognise it.

Following up our belief that you truly want to dazzle her, sweep her off her feet, stimulate her from every possible direction and take her to a completely new high, we offer here a collection of short but erotic stories. These you can read out loud, late on a winter afternoon with the curtains drawn against the dark, the sofa pulled up to the crackling log fire, the front door locked to outsiders and the room suffused with low light and warmth. If you possess a sheepskin rug, flaunt it. Put it on the ground before the fire and have your loved one snuggle into its deep pile.

MILDEST

(This was a short fantasy recounted by one of the members of Anne's sexuality groups).

SWIMMING

Linda pictures swimming in clear, blue water – the sea. 'The ripples of small waves waft past my shoulders, a breeze blows lightly on my face and the water streams past my body with every push of my powerful arms. The more I swim, the more powerful is the flow of the water under my body, across my breasts, and between my legs. The faster I go, the more I shiver with feeling. It flows and ebbs and flows again. I wonder and debate – if I come, will I drown?'

LESS MILD

(This was a second fantasy originally published in The Body Electric *by Anne Hooper (Pandora).)*

THE AUDITION

Dozens of men are sent up to audition for me. I am reclining on a couch, languidly watching them go through their paces. The purpose? To see who will have the immense good fortune to be my bed partner that night. A male secretary waits in the wings to usher in each new candidate, like a majordomo to Catherine of Russia. I dismiss one after the other with a curt 'Next!'

Finally, in comes an adorable – and very nervous – creature. I let him wait while I jot down a few brief impressions. This gorgeous man is dressed in very tight bleached-out blue jeans and a soft white shirt unbuttoned a little so that I can see the caramel-smooth skin of his chest. He has tiny hips and a lovely, small bottom outlined perfectly by the material of his jeans. I ask him to turn around, appreciating the play of muscles in his ropy thighs as he pivots slowly, and then I ask him to recite his vital statistics, including the size of his penis.

This makes him blush, but I am very businesslike. I order him to strip slowly. By the time he's down to his tiny black briefs, I have to admit that he's perfect. As he's beginning to peel them down, I call out sharply, 'I want you to lower them very slowly. Try to excite me – think about what you are doing.'

He tucks his thumbs in his briefs, inclining his pelvis slightly – rocking it in slight undulating movements – and teasing the material down a millimetre at a time.

First I get a glimpse of his curly, blond pubic hair, and then a tantalising view of the beginnings of his prick. He slips his hand down and allows his strong tapering fingers to caress the outer edges of his tense thighs, making cupping motions to emphasise and frame the swelling bulge.

'Very nice,' I say professionally. 'Before you show me what you've got, tell me what you'll do to me if you're chosen.'

Stammering, he tells me how much he wants to make love to me, to lick me from my toes to the nape of my neck.

Finally he pulls the briefs all the way down and his penis catapults out, fully erect and straining towards me – sort of pleading. I can see a pulse beating in his groin as he stands before me; a small groan escapes his lips and it looks to me as if his knees will buckle if I don't do something quickly.

'All right,' I say briskly. 'You've been selected. Be back at nine o'clock tonight.' Then he's taken off to the recovery room.

'Next,' I call out casually.

STRONG

(This short story was written for inclusion in this book. This and the next story are much longer and you may not want to read the entire episode in one session.)

TAKING RISKS

Sally and Tom were a terrific couple. Everyone agreed on that. Everyone of course was envious too. From their cute little basement flat, complete with white walls, stainless steel furniture and a ginger cat, Sally and Tom had it all. They earned, rumour had it, untold riches with, as yet, no children. Sally was a glossy brunette with clear, clear skin and a short geometric haircut. She favoured baggy clothes that hung elegantly on her slim body.

Tom was something in the city 'but not really a 'suit',' explained Sally to her friends. 'He's much too outgoing for that. Look at all the rugger he plays.'

It was true. One of the pre-requisites of the job was that you played rugby. The managing director captained the team and many an international deal had been done on the edge of the pitch, in the driving rain and churned up mud. Every weekend, come sun, snow or hurricane, the entire office turned out to battle with the elements and the other city brokers. Tom was short and wiry, and looked in fact, rather like his wife, with glossy dark hair that he wore unfashionably long.

Sally's educational qualifications were better than her husband's – a degree in German from the University of South Northumberland. But in her career as buyer for Cart and Tumbrell, an English chain store company specialising in, well, suits (although this time they were professional clothes for working women) she wasn't quite as highly paid as her husband. No matter. They earned well, saved well and were well on line for the next part of the life plan, which was to have children.

'How long have you two been together?' Sally's colleagues would ask, glancing admiringly at Sally's diamond Millennium ring and her holiday brochures for the South of Greece. It had been a while. It had in fact been 15 years and to tell the truth, although she wouldn't dream of doing so to her colleagues, it felt like a long time. It wasn't that she didn't get on with Tom. She did. They were remarkably in tune. They liked and disliked the same things, and were so in harmony that they hardly had to say a word to each other before they knew, so rewardingly, exactly what the other one was thinking.

And that was the trouble. They knew each other inside out. There were no surprises left. This was especially true when it came to sex. At least they still had sex – quite a lot of it considering how long they had been together. But it was always the same. Sally could calculate with precision timing just how long intercourse would take, what its pattern would consist of, which one of them would climax first, and which of them would have the loudest orgasm. This last amounted to a sociological phenomenon. Tom would have such explosive orgasms if his team had won that afternoon that Sally kept a special towel by the side of the bed to stuff over his mouth so that the neighbours wouldn't panic.

Recently Sally had surprised herself by feeling restless. It wasn't that sex with Tom wasn't good. It was. Remarkably so. Over the years the couple had refined their youthful congress to an art. Tom had even camcorded their activities once and the couple had gasped with smug delight when they viewed their own balletic movements on tape. Actually, watching that film had been the last time that Sally remembered feeling really enthusiastic about sex with her husband.

'No,' she mused, as she peered at a catalogue of Cart and Tumbrell's look-alike Armani suits, 'It's not that I don't like our life together. It's just that Tom has got really dull.'

She found her thoughts straying unconsciously back to this heretical realisation later in the week while she stood on the rugby touchline, jumping up and down in an effort to keep warm. Her revisiting of her newly awakened frustration may have had something to do with the fact that she had just walked past the changing room window and, glancing in, had seen one of the younger 'suits' without his suit. Being a rugby player, he'd looked remarkably athletic, muscles all in the right

place, buttocks pulled in just to the correct degree of hollow, a quick flash of tangled hair and six pack out front before he'd time to turn away to his locker.

'I'm aroused,' Sally murmured with surprise. The last time she had felt such unconscious stirrings was, well, when was it? For the life of her, Sally couldn't remember. Crossly, she pushed the thought to the bottom of her mind. There was no room for anything out of place in her life. She had no intention of getting led astray by an affair; she'd seen too many of her friends' relationships break up because of their lack of self-control. Sally was big on control. Every section of her life was positioned to perfection, each ornament exactly placed, her wardrobe colour-coded (she only wore oatmeal and pale yellow with a smattering of amber), her cat groomed every Saturday morning, her bowels moving at precisely 8am every morning. No, there was definitely no room for any spare member of the rugby team to intrude into her fantasy life. She was taking no risks.

At least, she would take no risks with anyone she knew. That way marital disaster certainly lay. But would the same risk attach to someone she didn't know? For the past few Sundays Sally had been browsing through the classified ads at the back of the Sunday newspapers – just for interest's sake, of course – and dreaming.

'Lonely bachelor millionaire seeks sexy female friend for mutual trips round the pole.'

Fat lot of good he would be, she'd figured at the time. The bachelor millionaire would probably turn out to be Tom's boss, who was undoubtedly rich but attached to a wife, three children, a pony and a dog and had a 47-inch waistline. All the same the idea had stuck. Not that the Sunday papers would help. The risk of meeting up with the man who lived next door was far too great. No, no, it really wouldn't do. Looking at her watch, Sally decided it was almost time for the tea break. She walked back to the clubhouse to unwrap the sandwiches from their clingfilm and trim off the outside crusts.

When the chaps had gone back out to play the second half, Sally and one of the other wives tidied up the kitchen. As Sally walked through the changing room to switch off the boiler, she noticed the mess. 'Probably wasting my time,' she grumbled as she piled empty beer cans and sweet wrappers into a black sack and stacked up piles of magazines neatly. But she tucked the mags to the back of the room where they wouldn't prove such a magnet. They were mainly of the girlie variety.

She was annoyed to see the pile wobble slightly. The glossies didn't fall but unable to bear a lurching stack, she removed the top layers to discover the cause of the trouble. This was a collection of much smaller magazines, which were unbalancing everything else. She placed them on top, shuffling them into place so that the sides rose in a straight line. That's better, she thought, stepping back.

Gazing out of the changing room window she decided against venturing on to the pitch again. It was truly arctic out there and the clubhouse was heated. Idly she picked up one of the magazines to kill time. And found herself riveted. She flicked through pages of dense type, pictures of naked women, gynaecological diagrams and close-ups (far too close) of genitalia. By the time she reached the back it came as a relief to discover a section with no lurid photographs, and no drawings of sex aids. Seizing upon it with haste, she subsided into the classifed ads. Thank God, they looked much like the ads in the Sundays.

At first glimpse they did indeed appear similar. There were still the millionaire bachelor variety but interspersed were others of very different tone. 'Vampire seeks stakeholder', read one. 'Christmas pudding seeks spoon and fork' went another. Fascinated Sally read on. There were literary references. 'Is there anyone out there who would play Abelard to my Heloise?' asked one hopeful. 'Leonardo di Caprio look-alike available for your very own scenario', caused her to pause and think. But no, she shook her head. Probably too young. After a while the small print dazzled her eyes and it was just as she was about the put the magazine down, that she saw it.

'Do you like everything in exactly the right place?' the advert ran. 'I do. Come and join me in getting straight.' She shook her head. This could have been written for her. The ad ended with a phone number. 'I'm not going to do anything about it, of course,' Sally said to herself. But just in case, (of what she wasn't quite sure,) she ripped out the ad, and popped it into her overcoat pocket.

The team won that afternoon and Sally found herself far too busy in the evening to give the incident another thought. But on Monday evening, when Tom went out to training, she remembered the piece of paper and transferred the phone number to a hidden recess of her computer. Perhaps it was the act of hiding it, perhaps it was just that the week was excessively dull, but Sally found herself going back in the following days to look at the number. She was nervous about replying

but one morning, in the office, her fears evaporated. Making such an enquiry would be like making any other call at work. All she would be doing would be finding out, for God's sake, what the advertisement was about. So she poked out the code on her Cart and Tumbrell own make of mobile and listened. 'Probably be an answerphone anyway,' she told herself. 'In which case I'll just switch off again.'

But a real live human answered her call. A youngish male, with a beautiful voice, sounding polite yet hesitant. Yes, he had placed the advertisement. What was he looking for? Well … There was a long silence and Sally began to think of ringing off.

He finally said, 'I suppose what I really want, if I'm going to be absolutely direct, is to make a new friend with the possibility of making love if that is what the new friend also wanted. How would you feel about that?'

How indeed? Sally found she liked his honesty. And she liked his voice, his manner. But she still had reservations. 'I would need a few safeguards,' she found herself saying.

'Of course,' he agreed. 'So would I. What are yours?'

'I am a private sort of person,' she said 'And although I think I like the sound of you, I need space and privacy. I wouldn't want to reveal any personal details.'

'No problem,' he said. 'I agree. We only ever meet by appointment and if we dislike each other at first sight we agree to be brave enough to say to the other person 'I don't think this going to work'.'

A ripple of relief ran through Sally. He sounded as if he might be all right. 'Where shall we meet?' she asked.

'Come over to my place,' he invited.

'You don't mind me knowing where you live?' she asked, surprised.

'Of course not,' he almost laughed. 'I'd like it, in fact.'

Later that week, Sally told Tom that she intended to go out to an exercise class on Thursday nights. 'It's another of your nights for training,' she pointed out. 'We'll be back at much the same time.

Seven-thirty, the next Thursday, saw her standing outside a small, newly painted front-door about two miles across the city. Smart square tubs containing bay trees were chained each side of the door and window boxes flowered with early blooming tulips, each bulb planted exactly six inches from the next.

The door was opened by a man of medium-height, aged around 35, with quite long, floppy dark hair and soft, brown skin. He had the kind of face that looked anxious until he smiled, when his entire features lit up. They lit up now. 'Come in,' he said. 'I'm so glad to see you,' and he pressed her hand in welcome.

She stepped over the Past Times front door mat and into a warm white interior, with white soft rug, white walls and white padded furniture. In the background tinkled harmonious New Age chimes, the aroma of coffee scented the air and the room was, well it felt exceptionally welcoming. It felt in fact as if Sally had known it all her life. She gave an unconscious sigh of relief and crossed the room.

Kicking her shoes off she sank into one of the generous sofas and beamed at him. 'What's your name?' she asked.

'You can call me David,' he suggested. 'And I,' he went on, 'will call you Hilary.'

Good, that suited her well. 'So what are the ground rules?' she asked.

'We have coffee together,' he said, 'and then make love. That is what you'd like, isn't it?'

It was indeed. Sally amazed herself by having no problem of any sort with David's lack of small talk, his refusal to beat around the bush. His openness, his directness about sex was attractive, quite seductive even. She looked at him and found herself picturing what he would look like naked. She liked what she saw. She liked the fact that she wasn't going to have to mess about making polite conversation. She adored the perfect symmetry of the walls, the angles of the furniture, the fact that David himself was clad in soft white tee shirt and cotton draw-string trousers. By remarkable coincidence she too had worn white that day. Her hands itched as she looked at his drawstring. She could see no discernible outline of underwear beneath. She flashed on to a sudden vision of David's soft naked flesh underneath the soft white cotton and for a mad moment, pictured herself diving headfirst into it.

'There's just one thing I think you ought to know,' she heard David saying. 'Before we start. It might make you change your mind.' She wrested herself away from the deep pores of his flesh with difficulty and prepared to give her full attention.

'I'm bisexual,' David told her. 'I have had, do have, partners of both sexes. I have been scrupulously careful about safe sex. I know I am completely clear of AIDs and if you feel at all worried about this, I can show you a recent letter from the clinic that confirms this.'

Sally hadn't expected this. She didn't know what to think.

Sensing her hesitation, he got out the letter and placed it on the steel coffee table. It was dated three days earlier. 'You'll have to take my word,' he added, 'that I haven't slept with anyone since then. But I haven't.' She found that she believed him. And smiled. Everything was going to be all right. And after that everything was.

The great thing was that he knew instinctively what was right for her. He held out his arms and invited her into them. He kissed her softly on the nape of the neck and plugged right into a nerve that sent her completely insane. Within seconds she was breathing heavily. And he, he had the sense to go on kissing. It was just when she thought she would expire from pleasure and he still hadn't moved from the magic spot when she suddenly had a thought – not a happy one.

'What about me?' She jerked away from him. 'You didn't ask about whether I had had an AIDs test. For all you know, I could have got it.' She was upset now. He stroked her comfortingly. 'I know,' he replied. 'Don't worry. I was going to talk about it. We won't have intercourse. We'll wait on that until you have had a test. I was going to suggest it after we had made love. You did seem in a bit of a hurry.'

That was true enough. She subsided. But she felt thrown off-balance, curiously upset.

'Look,' he showed her a peculiar little machine. Peering through an eyehole in a small cube she turned a handle on the side. Inside a woman appeared in close-up. As the handle turned the woman cunningly transformed into a flower, then blossomed with a bloom of petals curiously fashioned to look like female genitals. As the wheel turned, the woman, the flower and the genitals underwent a continuous cycle. Perhaps it was hypnotic, perhaps it simply took her mind off things but when she took her eye away from the peephole, she felt better. She also still felt aroused. He was OK. David was OK. Maybe she was mad to trust him. But she did.

'Come over to the rug,' He led her across the room to where a huge sheepskin was draped across a raised section of the floor. The section was soft, probably made of foam.

'Take my clothes off.' She helped him raise the white shirt over his shoulders and above his head. She placed finger and thumb on to the ties of the trousers and hesitated. Perhaps she would change her mind. 'Undo it,' said David. Suddenly she didn't really want to. But the man had said she must. Slowly, feeling like a child being asked to do something she knew was very wrong, she pulled at the string.

And was glad she had done so. David's skin was very tanned against the whiteness of the room. He stood out against it as if he were spotlit. Thoughtfully she folded his trousers into a neat pile.

The next half hour was perfect. David's love-making was art-work. With a wonderful body massage he skimmed his hands across her quivering body. He pushed her and pulled her, and tattooed her with fingertips; he scratched her softly; he sat across her prostrate body and swam his hands up and down her back in a sea surge of strokes. He stroked her down the side of the breasts, he stroked her on the inside of the thighs. He casually, oh so casually, allowed his hand to 'accidentally' brush against her labia. It was amazing just how 'accidental' that thigh-stroking hand turned out to be. And then, just as Sally waited breathlessly for the next 'accidental' brush, it didn't come. In fact he took his hands completely away from her body, folded his arms and did nothing.

After five minutes of silence she began to feel not only bereft of his touch but annoyed. What the hell was he playing at? After another five minutes of complete silence, with David sitting, silently waiting, Sally could contain herself no longer.

Seething she played down her anger. 'So what are you doing?' she asked, trying to appear casual. 'Oh, just waiting,' he replied. He was sitting with arms folded and legs in the lotus position.

'Waiting for what?' Sally was almost spitting, with annoyance and frustration and pent-up arousal.

He declined to say any more. Just folded his arms more firmly, sat there and waited. After a while Sally thought 'blow this for a game of soldiers', got up off the rug and walked angrily around the apartment. Still not a word. Sally started to pick things up off the window sills and crashing them down again angrily. Nothing. David looked for all the world as if he were practising meditation. She walked back towards the coffee table and picking up one of the immaculately positioned magazines there, dropped it deliberately on the floor. She did this with the second. And the third. Nothing.

Filled with anger, unable to bear the idea that she had somehow been made a fool of, and was now left high and dry, she began to kick the magazines viciously about the floor. Nothing. From out of her mouth erupted a low-pitched growl. 'How dare you,' she

snarled. 'How dare you make such a idiot of me. How dare you string me along like this, letting me think that you wanted to make love to me. How dare you be so bloody welcoming and then just shut me out as if I didn't exist, I didn't matter.' She paused for a minute and then 'And you can't even be bothered to reply.' She was screaming now, a deep low-pitch grinding rumble of a scream that shook the very bottom of her being and filled her body so tightly it was forced up out of her mouth and into the surrounding white space. She screamed and screamed and the white space became densely packed with her pent-up, long-suppressed, windings and grindings of physical desire transformed into rage. She screamed so long and so hard she was surprised the flat remained standing. She yelled and raged and gibbered and cursed, and wept huge hot tears which she dashed away angrily with a clenched fist. And yet he did nothing.

She cried and she wept, and sinking on to her knees felt completely hopeless, wasted, as if she'd run a long difficult race, pressed all her muscles into making a massive final burst and then been pipped at the post by a superior runner. Shaking all over she subsided into sobs and a heap on the floor. It was only as she lay there a muffled sob occasionally shaking her body that he moved. Walking over to her, he took her hand. 'Come over to the window Hilary,' he said. 'Now look out of it.' She looked and saw the view. It was a nice view, of the river, but what had that got to do with anything. As she looked, wondering what on earth she had bothered with any of this for, he softly rubbed her shoulders. His touch was oddly comforting. In spite of herself she relaxed slightly, leaning back against him.

'There, there,' he said reassuringly, and gathering her to him hugged her gently but caressingly from the back. It felt like being a little child after a terrible tantrum when your mother opened her arms and comforted you. With a huge muffled sob she turned and buried herself in his arms. For a while he rocked her, and stroked her and calmed her. After a while he turned her face towards his and kissed her very gently. She kissed him back, a drawn-out desperate, sucking, tonguing, longing sort of a kiss. She felt so hot, as if she'd had a fever. When he took his mouth away she couldn't bear it. Seeking after his lips she kissed him again this time urgently, needing him more than ever, desperate to clamp on to this man's mouth. The wonderful, amazing, joyous discovery was that he was kissing her back. And as he did so she was aware of his arousal. Very slowly, as if each movement corresponded to the passion that grew and grew between them, his penis became erect. Soon he was the one who couldn't let go. Soon he was the one who rather than stop kissing was biting her in his desire to make his mark, soon he was pushing her on to the floor, fighting to get at her, to get into her …

The next thing Sally knew was that his hand had jetted down the front of her body and was penetrating her as if it were his penis. He rubbed her and withdrew with the kind of rhythm his penis would have had if he'd put it inside her. He stroked and pushed, and bumped across her clitoris, and strayed around to the back and found regions there she had never dreamed could feel so alive, so on fire. Sally came and came and came again. She felt quite helpless in all this turbulence. This wasn't sex; it was being taken over completely; it was having no will of your own, no choice, no direction, only a flow of sensation so acute that for whole seconds she had no idea of where she was or what was happening, except that she was a mass of fire and molten sensation. And surrender. Yes, surrender. She would do anything for this man, go anywhere, behave outrageously if that was what he wanted.

Later, much later, Sally was stunned to discover that only an hour had passed. It felt like a lifetime. Will you come again Hilary? asked David, as he helped her get dressed.

'Do you want me to?' she asked, strangely unsure of herself.

'Yes, I'd like you to very much.'

Back home Sally was still shaking. 'That was a good workout,' commented Tom, looking at her flushed exhaustion.

'Yes,' said Sally absent-mindedly.

Love-making with David took on a pattern after that. A very satisfactory one. David had a way of putting ideas in your head, ideas that acted upon your emotions. Sally had never felt so complete in all her life. Sally found herself opening up to notions she would never normally have considered. David revealed to her, for example, the fact that he had another lover, also called Hilary, only this Hilary was a male. Oddly enough, Sally felt no shred of jealousy. Instead the thought of David and his two Hilarys filled her with erotic inspiration. When David eventually suggested that she might like to join him and the other Hilary in making love, she eagerly accepted.

She was the first to arrive that evening. She was keyed up, flushed with expectation, high on visions of these two bisexual men making love to her, both at the same time. When the doorbell rang a second time, David went to answer it. As he walked back into the huge living-room he masked the slighter man following him.

'Hilary,' said David, smiling at her, 'Meet Hilary.' He moved aside and the two Hilarys strode towards each other, hands proffered in greeting. And stopped abruptly.

'Tom?'

'Sally?'

'Oh,' said David, amused. 'Do you two know each other?'

STRONGER

(This short story was originally written for a collection of erotica.)

ARNO'S SEA CHANGE

It is the male who is expected to be the go-getter, the aggressor, the prime mover, the he-man who always directs the action in bed. The 'milksop' (who follows where his woman leads) is, by definition, not a 'proper' man. He isn't masculine, this has seeped away along with his status. There is little room in our deeply traditional society for males with passive natures.

But sex roles are changing baby. Women have got the bit between their teeth and boy, oh boy, does it taste good. Bother the 'new man' – a thing of the past – dead meat. What we babes in the 21st century seek is a paragon of magnetism – the feminine male – the *strong* feminine male. Anyone who caught the androgynous images of Queen, especially the amazing Freddie Mercury, when first tottering on to the record covers of the 1975s, knows exactly what I mean.

So I'll tell you the story of a man who crawled into my life and stuck like a burr in the corner. And when you hear about Arno, if I tell it right and if you listen with all your pores open, you'll get an inkling of the seeping pleasure of passivity.

Arno was a friend of a friend – one of those family connections people drift into and as often as not, drift out of again. Arno had the rugged face and deep tan of a regular guy, and by all accounts he was a good male, he'd done his duty as breadwinner and provider. Now, on the far side of a room crowded with friends, we look at each other across the Persian rug.

Deborah, his 11-year-old daughter, lies sprawled across his knee. As he looks at me, he is slowly stroking the back of her neck. Each of those unhurried strokes, fingertip light, is felt by me. His eyes transmit them and laser-like, their message burns into my flesh. A prickling heat floods up from the back of my neck. Judging from the emotions on his face, some strain of sensuality is correspondingly working its acid route to his pituitary.

This radioactive man has more sensual feeling in him than anyone else in the room. This man turns me on by thought. And no one else here knows anything about him. Not even his very beautiful wife. Discovering Arno is like finding the perfect pearl cast up on a reef of seaweed.

Arno was known to all of our party as the sexual cripple. He was the man with a weak character and a strange reluctance to go to bed. Arno was henpecked. He married a seventeen-year-old goddess yet never brought her to orgasm. Years of frustration later the goddess found another friend. She made no secret that she was forced to keep two husbands, one for companionship, the other for sex.

Occasionally, subterranean rumbles of protest would be heard from him. When the goddess went away on holiday with her lover and the children's nanny served Arno breakfast in bed that week, he consumed her along with the milk and cereal. The girl would lock the door of the bedroom behind her to prevent the children coming in as she waited on him. A gourmet holiday was had by all.

But the goddess fired her on return. That's when golf became the alternative to sex. Golf suited them both. It gave him something to do and her time off. Until I came onto the scene. I specialise in difficult people – I had married several of them. I hadn't wanted to fall in love with Arno; he didn't fit into my neat life at all. But apparently I needed a friend, for I found myself spending more and more time with him. We listened to poetry together, went to antique auctions, and revelled in country walks. It was the most beautiful country I've ever seen.

There was something about Arno's character that invited advances. My hands snaked out and made moves I never intended. I kissed and cuddled and hugged and snuggled without meaning to. You've heard of sleep-walking? This was sex-walking. With amazement, and delight, he responded.

I couldn't keep my hands away from him and, since he didn't seem to object, soon they travelled everywhere – everywhere that is except below the waist.

'Stop that,' he would order. 'I'm too sensitive.'

The wonderful hands I so admire today caressing his daughter then caressed me. But again his loving was all above the waist. His fingers and my fantasies were so in harmony that he had only to touch me on the ears or on the neck to give me orgasms. For me, whirling away up there in my erotic orifices, words became mundane. These auricular ecstasies sent waves of sweetness circling my body and lighting up my nerves. If you'd plugged me into an electrocardiograph the stylus would have drawn the pattern of a nuclear explosion.

The day came, the longed-for yet feared day. He showed up at the little apartment where I worked. Our fingers and lips were drifting like seaweed about each other before he got through the front door. My brain surged with Malibu breakers. Yet he did nothing he had not done before, a hundred times. And showed no signs that he would venture any further than he ever had.

I had other ideas. Quickly, deftly, I unzipped and stripped him. While he protested (mildly) I slipped off my own garments, leaving them just below the letter flap on the door mat. That only left his boxer shorts. I was now on fire, red in the face with possibilities. Kissing and biting him the long way down his torso I reached his sensitive abdomen. Skirting the taboo stomach I stroked and sucked and ran my nails along his hips and thighs. The mild protests changed to surprised cries of delight. Like the limbs of an octopus my tentacles snaked up his boxer shorts and quietly, casually, peeled them off.

'What are you doing?' Weak with delight, he didn't expect an answer.

Faced, for the first time, with my lover's penis, I grasped the reasons for my lover's less than lusty reputation, his quiet demeanour, his rumoured lack of sexual prowess. For he was small, that is to say not just small but minuscule – a micro male. Flaccid, he must have been one and a half inches long. And right now he was flaccid. Perhaps he was frightened of drowning.

Sweeping aside momentary doubts, I applied mouth to member resuscitation. Most men's penises are too big for my rosebud lips and hurt. But this, for once, was the perfect fit. Despite his agonised gasp, the quick clamp of hands over parts, the shame-faced turning away, I didn't hesitate. No one would stop me. And no one did. My power grew, my brain expanded, each vacuum sweep of my mouth intoxicated, super-tantalised. Each time my head rose smoothly on an upward swell, my vagina gasped; each golden flick and rainbow twirl of my tongue sent electrons of pleasure out through my body, tumbling over across the air and penetrating his. Slowly, reluctantly, his penis grew.

Time came when I arose from his genitals and looked at his face. His eyes were glazed with pleasure and his mouth sought mine quite blindly, like a new baby searching for the nipple. I pressed kisses into his cheeks, his temples, the sides of his mouth, before allowing his lips to fasten on to mine. Very deliberately my tongue rimmed the soft interior tissue and while he flooded with particles of pleasure, incapable of doing anything other than blindly receive, I slid my vagina on to his erection and enclosed him.

As I pulled up and away, I could feel his penis slipping wetly through my lips. As I bore down on him, my clitoris softly touched his pubic hair and diffused warmth and wetness. Each stroke brought slippery shoals of tropical dagger fish skirting around his penis and piercing his nerves in a thousand minuscule points. 'Keep still,' he begged. 'Keep still.' But I wouldn't. I drove him on, inflicting sensual abrasions in the slick between his body and mine, till goaded with an overload of driving, pounding, crashing storm, he broke. And collapsed, battered by sex, beneath me.

Which was just what I wanted. I licked my lips with vampire satisfaction, thrumming and vibrating, softly to myself. We lay together, we cuddled, we loved each other. And still I was thrumming. 'Now you've got to do something, Arno,' I thought to myself and began undulating around the man. He kissed me caringly. But remained still.

'Do I have to say something?' I asked myself. 'Do I have to break the magic spell and point out that I have needs too?' Perhaps the goddess never learned to speak out and so he never knew her frustrations till it was too late.

It sounded so easy to say, 'Arno, I want an orgasm. But terrified of spoiling the fantasy of our perfect rapport I dragged the words out from the interior of my gut.

He looked lost. 'But how?' he asked, pointing at his wilting flower.

'There are lots of ways, Arno.' There was no way I was going to let this once-in-a-lifetime, hit-by-the-thunderbolt love affair peter out.

'You're right of course.' He'd made up his mind. 'I'm lazy.'

'You are too good,' I impressed upon him, 'to let me leave you tortured by a surfeit of sexual excitement. You are far too good not to send my out of my skin with your lovely hands.'

He got the message. And for the first time in his life, dared to let his hands crawl down an electric female body. It wasn't difficult to get excited by him even though he'd never done this before. I didn't have to fake a thing. He hardly had to touch me down there before my cunt gasped and contracted with yearning. He felt me, rubbed me, lightly danced his finger-tips on the beacon of my sex and watched me avidly.

My body acted like it was on stage. If I had been faking, I would have been eminently theatrical. But my exaggerated tremors were for real. And he could see my reality and begin to understand what an aphrodisiac it is to be a powerful lover.

I cried out with every movement he made on my body, called his name in a language entirely my own. Inspired with the realisation for the first time that he was in total control of a woman, he substituted his mouth for his fingers. Although it sounds a slight fact on paper, it was a milestone in my impotent, miniature lover's life. He had acted purely from instinct. He'd done it because it had been wrenched from him by the hidden screams of my sexuality, so acute that they were out of the range of normal human hearing yet so insistent they impinged upon his cerebral cortex.

With each lap of his tongue, I climaxed out to a realm of fantasy, a science fiction range of orgasmic pictures. There was the sea of Earth frothing and boiling in a white ferment, there was the purple glow of the lichen-covered plant Mars, there were the wind torrents of Sirius where in a torture of iced fire, I scintillated in this fusion of mind and body.

It was the beginning of our addiction. From embracing open air, health and energy, we metamorphosed. In dark city streets at night, we'd huddle in doorways where I would hurriedly climb on to his penis. It didn't matter if I didn't come, I would be frisking his erection into helpless submission.

In the park, during the day, I'd force him to lie back, in the long grass, barely yards from the public path, my head bobbing over his penis, my hands torturing his balls. 'People can see,' he'd call in fear. 'You must stop.' But I wouldn't. I'd force him to climax before I would agree to continue the walk. In the park, at night, we'd pet in the car. 'Let's get in the back,' I would inveigle. And unzipping his fly I'd throw my skirt above my waist and bang him hard and mercilessly. Once, opening his eyes for a fleet second, he saw a peeping Tom, gazing jagged-eyed through the window. 'We must stop,' was Arno's instant plea. But I merely drove my white buttocks more menacingly through the air, refusing to let him go, shaming him with his public enthralment.

The culmination came when, weaving a tissue of lies, we escaped for a week to holiday to Spain. During the day he'd win golf championships while I would lie by the side of the pool. During the night, with the cockroaches scuttling through the bathroom, we'd make love. On the fifth day I felt hot and feverish. I couldn't eat so he left for supper without me. As my fever mounted, so too did my tumescence. Three times I relieved myself with sharp strokes of my fingers, seeing them as his cock between my legs.

He returned to me at midnight.

'Get on the bed.' It was the first time he'd ever ordered me to do anything. On the bed I rode him raspingly, deliberately causing accidents, making him fly in and out, catching him harsh and hurtfully in a tangle of genitals. Until he came.

I subsided on to his chest, waiting for his shrunken penis to fall out of me. It took its time. Finally, instead of moving out, it began to rub, softly, itchingly inside me. Unbelieving, I tested it a little, a trial pull along his length. He was still rigid. With each movement he grew until he was the size of a Tantric master.

'Turn over,' he commanded. On my back, in time-honoured female submission, I waited. Gently but firmly he sank deep into me. With each stop he bruised my clitoris. With each bruise the sensitive tissue spread until the wound haemorrhaged into climax. A soft, small spreading of orgasmic blood seeped sweetly through my loins.

Pausing for seconds, after my cries of pleasure, he looked at me eagle-wise. Pumping slowly, selfishly, at my moist membrane, his eyes closed as he climaxed into his prey. With a shudder we waited for his climax to end. But then, immediately, he began to move *again* inside me.

'Didn't you just come?' I questioned, puzzled.

'Yes,' he nodded. His clear green eyes met my surprise with amazement and pride. He continued moving. This time there was no change in his penis. If anything, it felt bigger and stronger than before. And this time when he moved he plunged into me as if he were punishing me for all the times I'd used him and forced him to perform.

'I'm going to fuck you,' he growled into my ear, 'until you can't stand up.' And pounding into me at one end he seized my ear at the other and raped it with his tongue. He forced the twisting wet tip inside and twirled it from lobe to drum. His hand stroked and scratched underneath my head and when he wasn't drowning my brain in a sea of static he bit me so hard around the mouth and the neck that he drew new blood.

Unable to control the reflexes of my churning genitals, spinning into confusion, my mind slipped into violently altered consciousness. There was nothing I could do to stop him whipping my cunt into pleasure and I spurted into shrieking, helpless, hurting delight. With a cry of victory he screamed into a third orgasm.

'Finally, I've had you,' he exalted. He was smug from satisfaction.

But then, so was I.

10

*d*KEEPING *esire* ALIVE

The one certainty is that everything changes. Sex is no exception. Sex never stays the same. Even if the lovemaking pattern sticks, the thoughts that accompany it drift and mutate. The urge for sex diminishes both with an individual partner and throughout time thanks to ageing. This doesn't mean that sex disappears or that it is less important. Most men and women want to feel that they will still enjoy the intimacy of bed and lovemaking in 20 or 30 years time. Ironically, to reach this utopia, you will (almost certainly) have to survive dozens of rows, rages, bouts of bad behaviour, downright drama, dishonesty and times when sex doesn't work.

Finding a way round these, hanging on to enough regard for the other to make a relationship worth retaining, simply surviving each other's differences are what love life is all about. Why do we even bother, when new partners can be so readily available? The simple answer is *attachment*. We become very attached to the people we love. To lose them is like losing a valued part of oneself. In losing a lover we injure ourselves. So, for self-protection alone, it's worth learning to overcome rage, to survive ill-feeling, maintain enough individual confidence to allow us to tolerate the other's temporary disapproval. And the sooner we can do this the better.

People are usually only too keen to get help when their relationship goes wrong. Yet few like the idea of working on a relationship *when things are going well*. If a relationship is worth having, they say, it should work spontaneously. You shouldn't have to think about it or analyse it. It should just be.

Alas, no. Relationships don't operate like that. There is always somebody doing the work in a relationship even if both partners are blithely unaware of this fact. What's more, even if you never verbalise it, you still possess expectations of a relationship. Should those expectations cease to be met, unhappiness seeps in, spreading poison.

What might such expectations consist of? Hof and Miller (1981) listed some of the long-term desires stated by couples taking part in enrichment programmes. These were:

- To promote awareness of the strengths and potential of growth of oneself, one's partner and the relationship
- The disclosure of thoughts and feelings
- To promote a partner's empathy and intimacy
- To improve couples' abilities to communicate, solve problems and resolve conflict

LONG-TERM SEX

Unfortunately no one seems to have carried out research on the link between sex and the survival of long-term partnership. This could be because the relevance of sex to couples' happiness is hard to quantify. Dr Jack Dominian (1979) stated that clinical experience taught him that, if sex didn't work well within the first six months of marriage, a type of emotional erosion occurred where each partner felt increasingly unlovable and unloved and grew increasingly unhappy. What Dominion is describing is the erosion of personal confidence. This is especially sad when the couple in question are good for each other in every other way.

To complicate matters further, although it sounds ultimately good sense to be able to foster trust, there are relationships where couples hardly know each other and yet the sex works well. And there are relationships where one partner is extremely angry with the other, the marriage is in a shambles and yet the sex continues to work brilliantly. Small wonder, then, that it's difficult to know where to start on keeping a good sex life alive and well. We are dividing this chapter therefore into two sections. The first section Making Relationships Work deals with marital behaviour and how to improve it. The second section Improving Sex focuses on the dilemma of trying to rejuvenate a jaded sexual relationship.

MAKING RELATIONSHIPS WORK

Marital therapist Dr John Gottman of the University of Washington has offered some important findings from 20 years work he has done with over 2,000 married couples.

He defines three specific types of marital style. These are:

- The validating marriage, where couples compromise often, calmly working things out
- The conflict-avoiding marriage where couples agree to disagree
- The volatile marriage that erupts often into passionate battles

Most people up till now have believed that the last two marriage styles are doomed for the divorce courts. But Gottman's long-term studies show paradoxically that this is not so. The reasons why? He has observed that, if the couples continue to offer each other a ratio of five good strokes to every one bad stroke, the marriage flourishes, despite conflicts. (By stroke here, we refer to the small but appreciative gestures that men and women use to make each other feel good. These may be verbal such as 'I love you' as well as physical, like hugging.) This is important information because it provides an answer to why some marriages successfully survive despite regular outbursts of anger.

GOOD STROKES

- Don't forget to say 'I love you' often and regularly
- Be appreciative – say thank you for small acts
- Buy small gifts to show that you care

THE FOUR HORSEMEN OF THE APOCALYPSE

Couples also need to avoid pitfalls. If you want to ensure the survival of your relationship you need to consciously steer clear of what Gottman calls the Four Horsemen of the Apocalypse. These are:

- Contempt

- Defensiveness

- Criticism

- Stone-walling

It is these hurtful and blocking behaviours that wound and drive lovers apart.

- Touch in small ways to demonstrate physically that you still want to stay connected emotionally
- Train yourself actively to show interest in what your partner says. Nod your head in appreciation, emphasise that you are listening by saying 'I see'
- When you feel happy, say so. This feels good to your partner
- Give compliments
- Tune in when you have upset your partner and apologise

CLUES TO BAD BEHAVIOUR

Followers of the Adlerian school of Individual Psychology believe that, as youngsters, we learn ways in which to relate to the world. How we learn depends on whether we have been encouraged or discouraged. If we are truly encouraged, we grow up to become emotionally balanced human beings. If we are discouraged, we devise unconscious methods of emotionally surviving. The theory goes that *all* attention-seeking has meaning. Bad behaviour isn't just bad behaviour. It's being done for a reason. Usually it's a plea to say 'please pay some good strokes into me'.

Individual Psychology believes that there are four main methods by which we show the degree of discouragement that we have reached. These are:

1 Attention-seeking

2 Trying to control others, bossing

3 Punishing or hurting others, seeking to revenge

4 Distancing or withdrawing

Each of these behaviours develops in childhood when we feel hurt or unwanted and each behaviour denotes a degree of emotional wounding or insecurity. Attention-seeking is, for example, the least wounded behaviour. Distancing is the most. Attention-seeking may be annoying but it is clearly healthier that trying to hurt others or becoming so depressed that you curl up into a ball and wish your partner would evaporate. These early childhood styles of behaviours provide a blueprint for how you are likely to react to significant adults in later life. That's the bad news.

The good news is that there are several methods in which such behaviours can be alleviated or reversed. For example, this is what you can do if your girlfriend starts to behave unhelpfully:

- Instead of rising to the bait, remind yourself that she is re-experiencing a childhood sensation of inferiority.
- Instead of coming back to her in *your* childhood mode (perhaps, mega-critically) operate on the bigger picture. See her for the hurt or discouraged infant she once was and offer her reassurance in the here and now. 'Yes, I can see you feel at a loss with this problem and don't quite know where to get results. But I am willing to try to improve the situation.' This will not only help the immediate problem, it will also start to reassure her in the long-term. *People can and do grow throughout the rest of their lives.*

Gottman's Four Horsemen of the Apocalypse (criticism, contempt, defensiveness, stone-walling) are negative behaviours that have been developed similarly as protective responses. What is useful about understanding why people behave in these negative ways is that you can begin to get a handle on your own behaviour. If, for example, *you* know that you automatically go into a criticism mode, which is a form of both control *and* revenge, you can learn to bite your tongue and say something positive instead. Once your woman friend understands that her attention-seeking, for example, is a throwback to an unhappy infancy and not necessarily indicative of the situation in the here and now, she can work on consciously altering her response.

IMPROVING THE QUALITY OF YOUR RELATIONSHIP

Should you find yourself bumping up against women like these, here are some methods of improving things:

Understanding
- Ask questions to understand or clarify.
- Hazard a guess to what childhood emotion lies underneath the present strong response.
- Paraphrase her thoughts or feelings in an attempt to get her to reveal more.

Negotiating
- Don't explode with anger – reserve that for another occasion.
- Show you have listened by nodding or asking pertinent questions.

- 💘 If you disagree do so courteously.
- 💘 Negotiate a trade-off. This means you may need to be prepared to make concessions of some sort but not to agree to do anything you know would be wrong or practically impossible to carry out.

Committing
- 💘 Agree to carry out a change.
- 💘 Make specific times or dates on which to do so.

Encouraging
- 💘 Bearing in mind that the woman behaving so badly before you is a very discouraged individual, offer her some form of appreciation or encouragement.
- 💘 Paraphrase her thoughts and feelings.
- 💘 Make empathetic statements.

FLOODING

John Gottman's research threw up the fact that men are in particular danger of 'flooding'. This overwhelming experience (that you are about 'to lose it' when an argument has gone 'too far') swamps men with dismaying rapidity. It's where real danger sets in. As a result of such flooding, people say and do things that they don't really mean, which always worsens the

MEN AND FLOODING

Gottman's studies showed that men's blood pressure and heart rate rose much higher and stayed elevated longer during difficult marital discussions than it did for their wives. He offers two theories to explain this:

- 💘 The first is that the male's autonomic nervous system, which controls the body's stress response, may be more sensitive and so men lose their tempers more quickly. It would also explain why women are apparently able to dive more readily than men into potentially difficult and dangerous discussions. They experience them to be far less threatening.

- 💘 The second is that men are more likely to dwell on the negative thoughts that keep them aggrieved. Instead of diffusing the situation, men are more likely to maintain their responses at a high level of aggression.

Gottman suggests that it is vital therefore for men to learn to calm down. As long as your system is flooded, it is impossible for you to think straight.

situation. Gottman believes in recognising when flooding is imminent and removing yourself from it until you've been able to calm down again.

Gottman suggests:

- 🐛 Taking a time-out. This means literally walking away from an arousing situation in order to calm down. However, to avoid making things worse with the partner, it's necessary to explain that this is what you are doing and that you will come back to the discussion when your pulse has steadied.

- 🐛 Deliberately work on methods of relaxing in the face of distress. Doing the tense/relax exercise (see Appendix B) all over the body so that you deliberately calm yourself physically.

- 🐛 When you return to the fight tell yourself firmly that this is only an argument and you can always move away again if necessary. And you do indeed have that freedom.

- 🐛 When arguing make a deliberate attempt to listen without leaping to your own defence. If this is hard, try an exercise called the Glass Window. As your partner rants, visualise a glass partition between the two of you, allowing you to observe her anger but also block off her rage.

- 🐛 This may feel hard to do but one way of taking the wind out of an angry partner's sails is by praising them. This works by reminding yourself that there are aspects of this person you like. By softening up your partner so that her anger is slightly diffused. You might ask her (nicely) on another occasion to do the same for you, in similar circumstances.

It's equally important to register that not only men are subject to flooding. Women are also capable of 'going over the top' given the provocation. When your woman does this with you, remember:

- 🐛 Let her get it all out before you attempt an answer. Even invite more so that she inevitably runs out of steam and feels as if her rant has been cathartic.

- 🐛 Make some offer of change but only something you can honestly carry out. The offer will help her feel she has been understood.

- 🐛 Carry out the change – so that she can see you take her seriously. She will then get to feel better.

ALTER YOUR STATE OF MIND

Later research (1999) supports Gottman's theory of 'flooding'. A team at Iowa State University subjected their human guinea pigs to extreme provocation. After being duly provoked, one group was allowed to go on and punch cushions before playing a computer game in which they could 'punch' a human opponent and generally demonstrate their aggression levels. The other group were told to sit quietly for a couple of minutes before playing the computer game. The second team proved less aggressive. By expressing all their anger, said Dr Brad Bushman, people were effectively practising being upset and this raised their discontent.

IMPROVING SEX

So far we've talked about improving the general *emotional* content of your relationship. But we've only done this on the grounds that good sexual relationships are dependent on the ability to talk, to negotiate, to feel comfortable in each other's presence and to feel trusting that when sex occurs, it will be in the best possible atmosphere.

Sometimes though, even when all these positive elements are present, sex still manages to heave a spanner into the works. For this reason we now look at ways to re-energise the hours you spend in the bedroom.

GETTING BACK INTO SEX

PARADOX

Invariably, when an activity is forbidden, you want it. The act of prohibition takes pressure off a situation and by placing something or somebody out of reach, the object or person grows more attractive.

ANXIETY

One of the difficulties in experiencing any kind of sexual slow down is that it sets up anxiety. Anxiety has a nasty habit of repeating itself on future occasions. Difficulties with impotence are a perfect example of this. Most men have a problem at some stage or other in getting an erection. *This is normal.* It's not a big deal. Or it shouldn't be a big deal. Unfortunately, we live in a culture that sets such unnatural standards that the occasional normal failure is seen as a disaster. A continuous stream of anxiety gets established as a result, which then sabotages the next attempt at sex. This is called the Performance Anxiety Cycle.

PARADOXICAL THERAPY

The therapy for the problem includes prohibiting intercourse and other activities leading to orgasm. This allows the sufferers to relax, feel more normal and then paradoxically, actively to want sex instead of dreading it. The same principle can be applied to improving the general quality of sex. If you or your woman friend are experiencing problems with any aspect of sex, suggest to her that you deliberately avoid going all the way for a while. *Tell her, as playfully as possible, that your body is not available, you positively forbid this anxiety-laden procedure!* The effect of paradox can then be joyfully felt.

SENSATE FOCUS

Paradox is not much use alone however. You also need to enhance the good sex that you've already got. This is where tried and trusty *sensate focus* is to be applied. This highly sensuous method of developing and expanding each other's tactility was devised by sex therapy pioneers Masters and Johnson and is used as the basis of all present day sexual enhancement. For one or two sessions a week, you are encouraged to set time aside in a warm room where you will be able to give each other caresses without interruption. For half an hour each, you take turns touching one other.

1 In this first session the touch is **expressive**. You are asked 'to talk with your hands'. The idea is that you express love and caring without words and that you do this through your 'expressive' touch. Any expressive kind of touch is allowed (kissing, squeezing, hugging, stroking) provided it is not sent or received as erotic. Sexual portions of the anatomy are out of bounds. Your partner may express her appreciation of your touch and you hers, but non-verbally this first time. 'Ums', 'ahs' and 'ohs' are all OK. *This expressive touching is for the benefit of the one doing the touching, not only the one being touched.* After about half an hour switch places and let your partner do the same. The toucher is the active participant, the partner, being touched, is passive.

2 In this second stage the expressive touch continues, although it may be expanded now to take in massage strokes if you chose. But now the partner does give specific **feedback**, albeit as non-verbally as possible. Assuming this is physically possible, the activity of 'hand-riding' can be included. Hand-riding consists of the passive partner's hand 'riding' the active partner's hand to suggest preferred speed, depth , direction, pressure, etc. This activity offers the open, completely non-pressured possibility of learning how each other may be pleasured. These affectionate, even passionate body strokes, can be a profound experience. (If they are not, this may be the sign that something else is wrong and that you might need some help from a therapist.)

3 This consists of more of the same but now the *breasts and genitals are included*. Intercourse is still off-limits. Obviously, the touch becomes much more sexual, offering opportunities for finding out what a partner likes within a still non-pressured atmosphere. The exercise evolves into a loving means of providing each other with explicitly sexual preferences that are both active and passive.

4 Continue to work in the same way but include **intercourse**. To begin with, the couple should opt for the woman-on-top position. Reminder: even now you are not aiming at orgasm. The object is to continue discovering each other's erotic sensation. If orgasm happens, despite yourselves, that's fine. But it is not the point of the exercise.

QUALITY TIME

In the stress and hustle of keeping afloat in a competitive world we forget that we need quality time together. In order for intimacy to flourish, time has to be set aside so that each can become sole focus for the other. Quality time is an agreement whereby the couple earmarks a certain period every week (a few hours can suffice) when they withdraw from the claims of friends, family, work and the telephone. The idea is to talk, touch, cuddle, go to bed together, do a massage, have sex, read aloud, have a bath together – whatever. The activity hasn't got to be sexual – the key principle is **scheduling** and **doing**. Committing to this exercise reinforces the belief that my partner 'loves me after all'.

IMPROVE SEX BY TAKING A BREAK FROM STRESS

Stress and overwork put huge strains on relationships and lay the groundwork for depression. To re-charge the emotional batteries, take small breaks at regular intervals and spend time in completely different places/environments.

SEX BOOKS

We've talked several times about reading together and the previous chapter even supplies erotic reading material to offer your woman something new. Reading matter, be it fiction or one of the many excellent manuals, can be thought-provoking, stimulate discussion and offer useful ideas about love-making. Some sex therapy courses make such books required reading and treat them as part of the therapeutic process. It is *not* however a good idea to thrust a sex book at a partner and say 'You've *got* to read this or we're doomed". That way she will feel criticised and discouraged. The best way to manage a reading assignment is to read the book yourself, and then offer snippets out loud. The more comments you relay like 'this is fascinating' and 'I never knew this before" the greater the likelihood of provoking curiosity and avoiding anxiety. If however, your partner suffers from an actual and specific sexual problem then there are several excellent books on women's sexuality (See Appendix C) from which you can gain practical solutions.

KEGEL EXERCISES

These are pelvic exercises that develop the muscle tone of the vagina in women and the penis in men. As a result of practising them, men develop ejaculatory awareness and control and women tone up the vagina so that orgasm is experienced with more strength and depth. The Kegels consist of voluntarily tightening then relaxing the pelvic muscles, which control the flow of urine. If this contract/relax exercise is carried out several times a day over a period of weeks, the vagina and the muscle at the base of the penis tone up like any other set of muscles.

MALE CONTROL

Women often (but not always) take longer to reach climax than young men. It can be difficult for you hanging on in there, waiting for her. The following might be helpful:

❣ Women are often not stimulated enough prior to penetration. So don't forget to excite her so much that she is desperate for you to enter into her *before* you go for penetration.

❣ But, if you are a quick-off-the-mark character, try training yourself *privately* prior to love-making. Use self-stimulation to get close to climax but then block ejaculation by firmly squeezing the penis between finger and thumb on the coronal ridge. If this is done hard enough (and don't panic, the penis can take extremely forceful squeezing without it hurting) the ejaculation subsides. So too may the penis but the next part of the exercise is to re-stimulate so that you learn to get erect again. You are effectively training yourself to believe that you can last longer as well as *actually doing so.*

- During intercourse, if you feel the 'point of no return' approaching, try the Beautrais Manoeuvre. Reaching round behind you, grasp your testicles and firmly pull them down. This blocks off ejaculation. You might try rehearsing this one as well.

- One way of learning to tolerate the sensation of being inside your partner's vagina is to have her sit on you during intercourse and move only enough to keep you erect within. This exercise is called the 'quiet vagina'. The object is to learn that you can cope with longer intervals of genital pleasure. Should ejaculation seem imminent either one of you can apply the squeeze.

- Combining these measures with methods of increasing your partner's ability to climax should go a long way towards matching up your orgasms. Ultimately though, as long as both of you manage a climax, it really doesn't matter in what order these happen or by what method!

TEN TIPS TO IMPROVE LOVE-MAKING

1 Understand what it takes to get *yourself* sexually aroused. Note and even write down the specific situations that seem exciting and arousing.

2 Understand what it takes to get your partner aroused. Note down specific situations and conditions that turn *her* on.

3 When you are not aroused, try love-making in ways other than sexual intercourse. Expand your horizons. Get to know alternative ways of getting close. Intercourse isn't the only pathway to great sex.

4 Encourage your partner to tell you what she likes. Hear her suggestions with calm and acceptance. Work on doing this through the medium of touch.

5 Increase touching in your relationship generally. Feel happy about doing so and understand that touch can be directly related to the growth of trust and desire.

6 Become an excellent lover without using your genitals. Be affectionate and caring without expecting intercourse.

7 Don't try to force your partner's response. And take care you do not get your sexual identity from your partner's response.

8 Let arousal be something that grows between you. Don't always approach your partner physically with the goal of having sex.

9 If you've been together for several years don't expect your partner to always be aroused every time. Expect to take turns in initiating sex.

10 Make your partner the focus of your loving. 'Who' is more important than 'how'.

GENERATING INTIMACY

Intimacy is a kind of amalgam of love and sex. Men and women tend to miss the loss of intimacy more than they do that of sex. If you have lived together for some years perhaps there isn't such a personal feel about the relationship. Perhaps you regret this and long to inject something energising into the relationship to restore intimacy once again.

The key to generating intimacy is to move in your partner's direction. The very act of doing so implies warmth, curiosity, some desire. However, movement is not enough – you have to offer a lover what she really wants. Altruistic giving, the sort that counts, must come from an overflowing desire on your part to give. In order to do this you need to feel that *she* is sincerely paying attention to who *you* are and what *you* want. In other words, the ingredients of intimacy are circular. They are a true spontaneous exchange of appreciation and admiration.

Just because it's spontaneous doesn't mean that we can't also think carefully about the process. When we give, it's helpful to give not what we think *we* would like, but what we suspect *she* would like. That's because if you really care about someone you put her first, because you value her so highly.

This can be surprisingly scary to do. Getting what we want in the way of love and intimacy sometimes frightens us to death. When someone has longed for love, attention and intense closeness, then finally gets it, this can arouse all kind of feelings of anxiety and grief. Love and Brown (1999) say that there's a reason for it. 'The end of longing is the beginning of grief. It's called 'reunion grief',' they write. 'When people are longing and yearning for love, they are holding at bay the grief of not having had the love they've needed. Therefore getting that love is terrifying and painful, full of angst – but worth the price of feeling it.'

Please don't panic. Not everyone feels such pain when they are at their most joyful and it has to be remembered that Love and Brown are marital counsellors (from Austin, Texas) who see some of the casualties

BASIC BODY MASSAGE

❧ Basic massage strokes for the whole body are circling with your hands moving in small circles, palms down on your partner's skin, always massaging away from the spine.

❧ A general rule is not to massage bony areas, to start with a firm pressure and as you want to increase the erotic sensation, to lighten the pressure.

❧ The most erotic pressures of all are fingertip massage and even fingernail massage.

❧ Hands should always be warm, it's best to use a good massage oil and above all, make the strokes extremely slow, the slower the better.

of strong emotions. They make some interesting observations however about intimacy and passion. Intimacy, they expound, is not just the prelude to passion, it's the precondition. 'Without the component of intimacy there will be no passion. To know and be known by another and live in connectedness is erotic. Libido means literally life energy. To combine this spirituality with sexuality is an altered state'

Assuming that you and your lover are nearing that joyous altered state here are a few moving and powerful touch routines to bring tears of happiness to her eyes. Anne Hooper writes: 'When, years ago I was learning massage routines with massage master Ray Stubbs of San Francisco, there was one advanced touch exercise seen as a reward for doing well. It is incredibly sexy to give and even better to receive.

'Peacock feathers, fur gloves, a warm bath, a hot towel and an erotic massage that lasts for hours sound like elements from some fantastic dream. But these were all elements of the wonderful treat that I experienced at Ray's hands.

'Ray began by telling me a wonderful story while I lay resting on a comfortable mattress. He encouraged me to picture the scenery on a wonderful beach and I saw it as the beach on an alien moon glowing with colour. Afterwards Ray played a little soft flute music as I continued to lie, perfectly relaxed. He had already bathed me in warm soapy water and towelled me dry with hot fluffy towels, refusing to let me do any of the drying myself.

'Once I was fully at ease he commenced to give me a wonderful sensual massage. He started by stroking my skin with velvet, then fur, then peacock feathers. When he graduated to his hands he started at my back, moving on to my front, taking in my arms and legs and eventually moving on to my genitals. All good sensual massages start with a whole body massage – it is never a good idea to neglect the rest of the body and focus only on the sexy bits. Ray never expected or wanted any sexual reward for these treats.'

RAY STUBB'S INTIMATE MASSAGE FOR WOMEN

Gentle Hair Tease: Don't think twice about it and don't question this instruction – just begin by pulling her pubic hairs, almost one by one, very gently and very slowly. Work your way from the top of the pubic triangle, right down to the hairs on each side of the labia between her legs. Take a long unhurried time over this and we promise, you'll be appreciated.

Drowning: Take a bottle of warm massage oil in your let hand. Slowly and carefully pour a little of it over your right hand shaped with the fingers pointing downwards and together, looking a little like a duck's bill. The object of this is to allow the oil to seep slowly through your fingers and down your fingertips so that it runs on and down her genitals. It feels, to the woman, like a safe flood of warmth. (Now you can understand the necessity for the oil to be gently heated. Flooding with cold oil is a nasty experience. The best way to heat the oil is to float the bottle in the bath at the start of an evening.)

Pulling: Separate the outer lips of the vagina from the inner and, with both hands on one outer lip, gently pull and let go, pull and let go, in a rhythmic pattern, starting at the very end of the lip away from the clitoris and working up the lip towards the clitoris. A good analogy for this movement is the kind of lip-pulling a child sometimes does on her mouth to make funny little flapping sounds.

You could pull the lip perhaps half a dozen times or more on your journey up. Then repeat, very gently, on the other side. Then repeat with a hand on each lip at the same time. Do the same with the inner lips, starting with first one, then the other, then both at the same time.

You may need to separate the inner lips when you begin but it is quite likely that your partner will have become aroused. If this is the case, her labia will have swelled a little and naturally separated. The inner lips usually meet over the clitoris, forming the clitoral hood and when you reach the clitoral end make sure that you continue the act of 'pulling-and-then-letting-go-gently' over the clitoral hood as well.

Circling: With the forefinger, carefully and sensitively run your finger around and around the clitoris, never touching the top, simply circling and circling. After a dozen or so circles change the stroke to rubbing lightly up and down on the left side of the clitoris a dozen times, then on the right side of the clitoris a dozen times. Still with the forefingers, rub backwards and forwards immediately below the clitoris a dozen times and then from the clitoris down to the opening of the vagina and back, also a dozen times. Men tend to think women prefer clitoral stimulation to be firm and direct, but this isn't always the case.

The energy sweep: Most women are so aroused by genital massage that the obvious move to make next is to go on to mutual lovemaking. Just in case she doesn't want to do this but is still very aroused, a good way of diffusing the sexual energy you have created is as follows. Hold out your hands flat, about an inch above your partner's body (like a hovercraft) and 'sweep' the energy that the body radiates out of the hands, the feet and the head. You don't need to actually touch your partner in order to do this. Just skim your hands above their body as described. A surprising feeling of completion is reported when massage is terminated this way.

RAY STUBBS' ULTIMATE MASSAGE

This is a massage technique that Ray only teaches to couples for reasons that will rapidly become obvious. He calls it the Three-Handed Massage. Ray suggests starting with a 15 minute regular massage so that the whole body is warm and glowing. Then, he writes: 'With your partner lying face down, help her to relax by massaging her back.'

The idea is to coat her back with slippery oil and after stroking and caressing her to sit astride her thighs and buttocks. At this stage, you coat yourself with oil, on the abdomen, genitals and thighs. Then leaning forward let yourself gently slide along her body, as you continue to stroke, caress and massage her back. Ray suggests it should be like 'slow dancing, swaying to the music in the background'.

Gradually, as you move and flow along her body, up and down, let your penis slowly, imperceptibly, enter her vagina. Allow yourself to flow along and inside her body so that she is being massaged three ways, by your two hands and by your erect penis from within. Try and slowly massage as many parts of her body as you can reach from this position, you may even be able to get your hands down to the calves of her legs.

After a long time of this rocking, floating massage invite your lover to turn over. Then carry out the same exercise from the front. It doesn't matter if it doesn't end in climax, orgasm is not the object of the exercise. What you are aiming at is giving her a complete sensual massage where every inch of her body feels loved and cherished. Nor does it matter how the massage ends. The important thing, Ray advises, is to linger. Let the rosy glow of massage continue for as long as possible. Enjoy, enjoy.

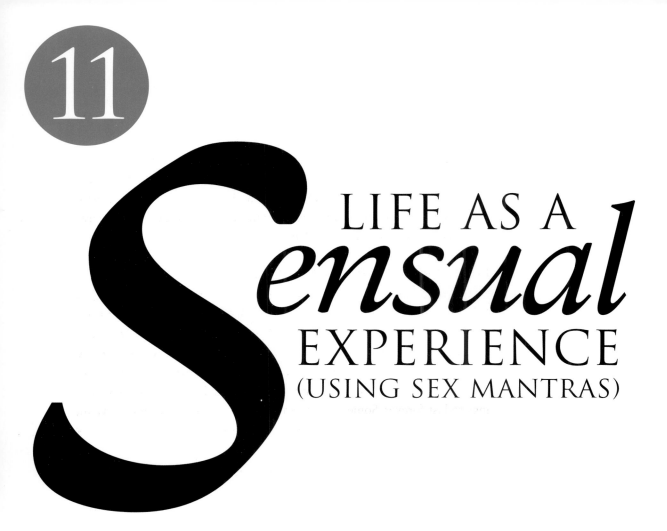

11

LIFE AS A *Sensual* EXPERIENCE
(USING SEX MANTRAS)

You will have read this book for a number of reasons. Your may have been feeling apprehensive about your powers to be a good lover. You may have been seized with ambition about a particular woman on whom it was vital to make a profound impact. You may simply be curious about sex along with the rest of the race.

In this book we hope we have offered you routes to good sex by way of love. Lovemaking isn't just about 'left hand down there, George'. Because we don't believe in making sex mechanistic we intentionally describe therapy routines offering *touch with feeling*. The sensate focus exercise found in the previous chapter is the later version devised by Masters and Johnson after they realised their original was too clinical. This revised version is about expressing through your hands what the rest of your mind and body is longing to pour out.

Equipped with the skills we have described so far there is just one further ingredient you'll need before you become a fully confident maestro of the bedroom. It's a philosophical outlook. It's an understanding that some relationships naturally go well and others do not. It's the equilibrium to enjoy a wonderful love and survive the transformation of passion to something tender but less dramatic. It's a link between wanting to be a great lover and understanding that you live in the 'here and now'. Are the authors losing their marbles? How can you *not* live in the here and now? We'll explain.

LIVING IN THE HERE AND NOW

In our increasingly pressured world, it is good to value what you enjoy. It is a correspondingly bad idea to let yourself get gloomy by constantly predicting what *might* go wrong and what you *might* lose. In a love affair, it's especially important to avoid this because the state of wanting sex every night, for example, rarely lasts for more than about six months. This is utterly dismaying since we long for these amazing feelings to last forever. Sometimes when a great relationship goes long-term, we puzzlingly experience a disappointment or grief. It isn't perfect any more. Why should this occur?

The ridiculously simple answer is that, by mere virtue of being alive, we change and relationships change. We don't have to do anything special to create the alteration. All love affairs are turning into something else, and all excitement gets partially burned up.

We are constantly gathering new ideas, behaviours, habits, sensations, chunks of information and satisfying our curiosities. Every time this occurs we modify our beliefs and re-direct our feelings. Such transformational change can be helped by not digging in our heels *but following the flow* (since its force is ultimately irresistible).

This doesn't mean that we can't steer ourselves in a preferred direction. Indeed, that's where this book comes in. But the current cannot really be reversed, whether you mean the currents of time, or ageing or the knowledge you gain through experience. We hope that by reading this book you can re-make some of your ideas of how you want to be with your lover and how you might best go about establishing a better and greater loving.

VISUALISE LIFE POSITIVELY

Now is the time for a positive outlook. Now is the time for deliberately focusing on the gains of the here and now. The future has not yet happened. The present is with us, we live in it and are fully able to modify our attitudes towards it. You might therefore think, this about your lover:

❧ She is lovely. I feel special to have known her and to continue knowing her.

❧ I enjoy most of the time I spend with her.

❧ By knowing her, I have been changed and I have changed her.

❧ The greater knowledge I acquired through knowing her will stand me in good stead in continuing to love and regard her.

By thinking like this, we acquire a sense of peace during the process of change. The inexorable journey of the love affair stops being threatening and turns into one of discovery.

PLAYING WITH DIFFERENT VERSIONS OF REALITY

Psychotherapist Emmy van Deurzen-Smith says that it can be enormously freeing to recognise that all human experience is composed, in part, of interpretation. There will be many different interpretations for one event. The author Lawrence Durrrell wrote a quartet of books around this principle. Each book told the same story through the eyes of a different character. Each story sounded unique. This means that while your experience of your love affair is specially yours, it also means that there are many other ways of seeing it. Once you can take that idea on board there are innumerable systems for valuing life. Some of these may offer you a new appreciation of yourself.

❧ You might be able, for the first time, to discover how much a partner values your loving as well as your sexuality.

❧ You might enjoy aspects of yourself you didn't previously know existed because she has seen them in you.

All of these less dramatic, but more profound experiences, feed the inner craving to be loved and valued.

VALUE EVERYDAY BEAUTY

As you walk through the streets, look about you. Actually see what you are passing. How often do you really take in the shape of a lamp-post, the green of lawns or fields, the warmth of your grip on your partner's arm? To be alive is to be full of good things. Stop right where you are as you read this. Reach out and touch whatever object is nearest. Take a long hard look at it. And next time you feel remotely down, deliberately do the same.

Some people find this harder to do than others. We think now that is because they may have experienced a lack of love and warmth during childhood leaving a sense of incompleteness deep inside. Yet human beings, as the philosopher Sartre pointed out, tend to notice what they lack. The remedy is to turn the feeling on its head and see how much we possess as well. A glass half empty still contains a satisfying and refreshing drink even though half the contents may be missing!

These ideas may surprise you. They are probably not what you expected to find in a sex book. Yet sex goes through many transformations. In order to continue valuing the strength and depth of a good sexual relationship *through time*, we need to expand our minds. We need to see that there will *always* be something of value, even on the occasions when we may not immediately feel it. This isn't easy to do. One problem is that we get held back by the belief that because we are thinking and behaving a little differently to our friends we will be laughed at. Yet innovators are people whose ideas often don't fit in with current thinking. This doesn't prevent those ideas sometimes from becoming of immense value. In fact, it's amazing how a firmly held belief can end up influencing others. First one person then a second accepts your newer way of valuing relationships and before you know it whole swathes of the population follow suit.

So living in the here and now means being sensitive to the woman you love but unafraid of your own desires and enjoyment. If a relationship doesn't go well, learn from your mistakes and try again. In order to avoid depression, always look for what you have enjoyed and what you have gained. Put negative thoughts firmly out of your mind. Try re-framing the situation you see yourself in *positively* and move on. Understand how fortunate life is. *Your* life.

MANTRAS

Mantras are simple phrases that act as reinforcers of intent. The purpose of a mantra is not to chant it as a meaningless mumble, or Californian revelation, but to think about it and spur yourself to act on it. One young woman who had been suffering from depression was given the mantra 'I am free to be joyous'. She carried it about with her at the front of her wallet so that every time she opened the wallet to get out banknotes, the message appeared before her eyes. When a few weeks later she nervously found herself about to be kissed by someone, she remembered the mantra and told herself that 'it was all right to be kissed' and 'it was all right to enjoy it'.

She found herself enfolded in the most sensual experience she had known for years and her chemical reaction to the kiss zapped right down to her boots and back. Afterwards, her depression lifted, her friendships improved and her work went from strength to strength. Coincidence? Who knows!

On the grounds that we should all keep open minds and look for the best within ourselves we offer here suggestions for a few mantras that may assist your enjoyment of life and love.

I APPROVE OF MYSELF

I AM FREE TO BE LOVING

I AM HAPPY WITH MY SEXUALITY

I CHOOSE TO ACCEPT SENSUALITY FREELY AND FLEXIBLY

I AM LOVING AND ENDURING

I RECOGNISE MY BODY AS A FOUNT OF SEXUALITY

I AM SAFE TO BE MALE

I ACCEPT AND REJOICE IN MY MASCULINITY

I AM TOTALLY CONNECTED TO LOVE

I SING THE JOYS OF LOVE

I AM THE LIVING, LOVING EXPRESSION OF SENSUALITY

I AM BALANCED IN MY SEXUALITY